Radiology Life Support (Rad-LS)

A practical approach

EDITED BY

William H. Bush Jr MD FACR
Professor of Radiology, Director, Genitourinary Radiology,
University of Washington School of Medicine, Seattle, Washington

Karl N. Krecke MD
Assistant Professor of Radiology, Head, Section of Neuroradiology,
Mayo Clinic, Rochester, Minnesota

Bernard F. King Jr MD
Associate Professor of Radiology, Abdominal Imaging and Genitourinary Radiology,
Mayo Clinic, Rochester, Minnesota

Michael A. Bettmann MD FACR
Professor of Radiology, Dartmouth Medical School,
Chief of Cardiovascular and Interventional Radiology,
Dartmouth-Hitchcock Medical Center, Lebanon, New Hampshire

A member of the Hodder Headline Group
LONDON • SYDNEY • AUCKLAND
Co-published in the United States of America by
Oxford University Press Inc., New York

First published in Great Britain in 1999 by
Arnold, a member of the Hodder Headline Group,
338 Euston Road, London NW1 3BH

http://www.arnoldpublishers.com

Co-published in the United States of America by
Oxford University Press Inc.,
198 Madison Avenue, New York, NY10016
Oxford is a registered trademark of Oxford University Press

While the advice and information in this book are believed to be true and accurate at the
date of going to press, neither the author[s] nor the publisher can accept any legal
responsiblity or liability for any errors or omissions that may be made. In particular (but
without limiting the generality of the preceding disclaimer) every effort has been made to
check drug dosages; however, it is still possible that errors have been missed.
Furthermore, dosage schedules are constantly being revised and new side-effects recognized. For these reasons the reader is strongly urged to consult the drug companies'
printed instructions before administering any of the drugs recommended in this book.

British Library Cataloguing in Publication Data
A catalogue record for this book is available from the British Library

Library of Congress Cataloging-in-Publication Data
A catalog record for this book is available from the Library of Congress

ISBN 0 340 74158 9

2 3 4 5 6 7 8 9 10

Commissioning Editor: Nick Dunton
Production Editor: Wendy Rooke
Production Controller: Sarah Kett
Cover Design: Mouse Mat

Typeset in 11/13 pt Goudy by Saxon Graphics Ltd, Derby

What do you think about this book? Or any other Arnold title?
Please send your comments to feedback.arnold@hodder.co.uk

Contents

List of contributors

William H. Bush Jr MD FACR
Professor of Radiology
Director, Genitourinary Radiology
University of Washington School of Medicine
Seattle, Washington

Karl N. Krecke MD
Assistant Professor of Radiology
Head, Section of Neuroradiology
Mayo Clinic
Rochester, Minnesota

Bernard F. King Jr MD
Associate Professor of Radiology
Abdominal Imaging and Genitourinary
    Radiology
Mayo Clinic
Rochester, Minnesota

Michael A. Bettmann MD FACR
Professor of Radiology
Dartmouth Medical School
Chief of Cardiovascular and Interventional
    Radiology
Dartmouth-Hitchcock Medical Center
Lebanon, New Hampshire

Thomas F. Bugliosi MD
Consultant
Department of Internal Medicine
Division of Emergency Medical Services
Mayo Clinic
Rochester, Minnesota

Richard H. Cohan MD
Professor
Department of Radiology
University of Michigan Hospitals
Ann Arbor, Michigan

Geoffrey S. Ferguson MD
Clinical Associate Professor of Radiology
University of Washington School of Medicine
Interventional Section
Department of Radiology
Northwest Hospital
Seattle, Washington

Daniel G. Hankins MD FACEP
Consultant
Emergency Medical Services
Mayo Clinic
Rochester, Minnesota

Jane S. Matsumoto MD
Assistant Professor
Section of Pediatric Radiology
Mayo Clinic
Rochester, Minnesota

Jeffrey P. Quam MD
Assistant Professor
Department of Diagnostic Radiology
Mayo Clinic
Rochester, Minnesota

Henrik S. Thomsen MD
Professor of Radiology
Department of Diagnostic Radiology
Copenhagen University Hospital at Herlev
Herlev, Denmark

John T. Wald MD
Section of Neuroradiology
Mayo Clinic
Rochester, Minnesota

Preface

Radiology Life Support (Rad-LS): A Practical Approach is the culmination of the efforts and contributions of many individuals. The concept of comprehensive training in the treatment of reactions to radiographic contrast materials and other emergencies was developed by Geoffrey F. Ferguson MD, an angiographer and interventionist at Group Health Hospital in Seattle, Washington. In the late 1980s he realized the need to train radiologists and radiology personnel formally in the recognition and treatment of adverse events unique to the radiology department. Coordinating contributions from radiology, anesthesiology and emergency departments, he organized a course covering contrast reactions as well as airway management and early defibrillation. One of the strengths of Dr Ferguson's concept was the interactive format in managing sample cases by selecting correct medication, discussing options for airway management, and identifying cardiac dysrhythmias and appropriate application of defibrillation. In subsequent years, William H. Bush Jr MD, from the University of Washington, joined the course faculty.

Bernard F. King Jr MD, Karl N. Krecke MD and Sherrie L. Prescott RN, all from the Mayo Clinic's Department of Diagnostic Radiology, attended Dr Ferguson's course and adapted it to teach residents, staff radiologists and nurses in Rochester, Minnesota. They expanded the format to include small-group sessions stressing the management of contrast reactions, airway and basic defibrillation, utilizing emergency scenarios and one-to-one faculty–student interaction. The success of the course led to presentation to other Minnesota radiologists, and subsequently nationally at selected Mayo Clinic meetings.

From these beginnings, and under the guidance of Drs King, Bush and Krecke, evolved a Radiology Life Support (Rad-LS) course that was presented in 1995 at the American Roentgen Ray Society (ARRS) Annual Meeting. It has been heartily endorsed by attendees as addressing the needs of radiologists and radiology personnel in the community who are confronted with adverse reactions to injected contrast media, particularly unexpected severe reactions. The Rad-LS course continues to form part of the annual ARRS meeting. The main principles of the course are active participation by the radiologist and other personnel in quickly and accurately identifying the type of adverse reaction, choosing a course of action, and instituting therapy from a small group of effective medications. Basic airway management and appropriate use of early defibrillation are also taught. This book has, in turn, evolved from the Rad-LS course and syllabus.

Radiology Life Support (Rad-LS): A Practical Approach focuses on the recognition and treatment of emergencies that occur in the radiology department. The identification, initial approach, principles of treatment, and selection of specific therapeutic measures reflect our combined experience. We believe that the contents constitute practical and effective applications of the science and art of managing radiological emergencies.

The book begins with the important topics of intravascular contrast media biochemistry and physiology, presentations of contrast reactions, specific treatment of reactions in both adults and children, and airway management in adults and children. An extensive resource chapter on cardiac dysrhythmias, their management, selected drugs, and basic algorithms for dealing with acute life-threatening cardiac events completes the initial chapters dealing with emergencies. As more technically complex imaging studies and interventional techniques have developed, so has the need to provide sedation and manage pain, and these principles and the specific drugs for both children and adults are reviewed. Discussion of the use of contrast media in radiology would not be complete without specific information on the management of contrast extravasation and the problem of contrast-induced nephrotoxicity. Finally, there are complementary case studies.

It is the hope of the editors and authors of this book that, when an emergency event occurs in your department, you will now have the knowledge and expertise to act quickly and effectively to the optimum benefit of your patient.

William H. Bush Jr MD, FACR
Karl N. Krecke MD
Bernard F. King Jr MD
Michael A. Bettmann MD, FACR

Acknowledgments

As indicated in the Preface, the initial efforts and continued support of Dr Geoffrey F. Ferguson are noteworthy.

Special thanks are due to B.J. James, secretary to Drs King and Krecke, for her tireless efforts in organizing and coordinating the Radiology Life Support course and the initial syllabus used for that course.

We also thank Drs Joseph T. Ferrucci Jr and Albert A. Moss, past presidents of the American Roentgen Ray Society, who advanced our goal of educating our colleagues in radiology, Dr Bruce L. McClennan, Chairman of Refresher Courses of the American Roentgen Ray Society (ARRS), who recognized the need and made it happen, and Susan Roberts and her staff at the ARRS for the support they have given us in presenting the initial and subsequent Radiology Life Support courses.

William H. Bush Jr MD, FACR
Karl N. Krecke MD
Bernard F. King Jr MD
Michael A. Bettmann MD, FACR

Intravascular contrast media and premedication[*]

Bernard F. King Jr

Historical perspective

Iodinated contrast media were first recognized and utilized in the 1920s, after researchers at the Mayo Clinic noted bladder opacification on abdominal radiographs in patients who had received intravenous sodium iodide for the treatment of syphilis. Because of this serendipitous discovery and because of the unique X-ray absorption of iodine, much investigation followed into developing a safe iodinated intravenous contrast medium.

The first relatively safe iodinated contrast media were introduced in the 1950s. These agents were basically tri-iodinated benzene rings with organic side-chains in the 3 and 5 positions of the benzene ring (Fig. 1.1). A carboxyl group was added in the number 1 position which improved water solubility. This carboxyl group dissociated into a cation (H^+) and an anion (the benzene-ring complex). These agents are called ionic agents because, when they go into solution, they dissociate into an anion and a cation. In the late 1980s, nonionic iodinated contrast media were introduced (Fig. 1.2).

Similarly, the first intravenous gadolinium-based contrast media were introduced in the late 1980s (Fig. 1.3). Recently, organ-specific MR contrast and intravenous ultrasound contrast media were introduced.

Classification

The classification of iodinated contrast media can be made from many different perspectives (e.g. ionic vs. nonionic, low-osmolality vs. high-osmolality, monomers

[*]From King BF Jr, Krecke KN, Prescott SL (Course Directors): *Advanced Radiology Life Support*™ (ARLS). © 1998, reproduced with permission of the Mayo Foundation.

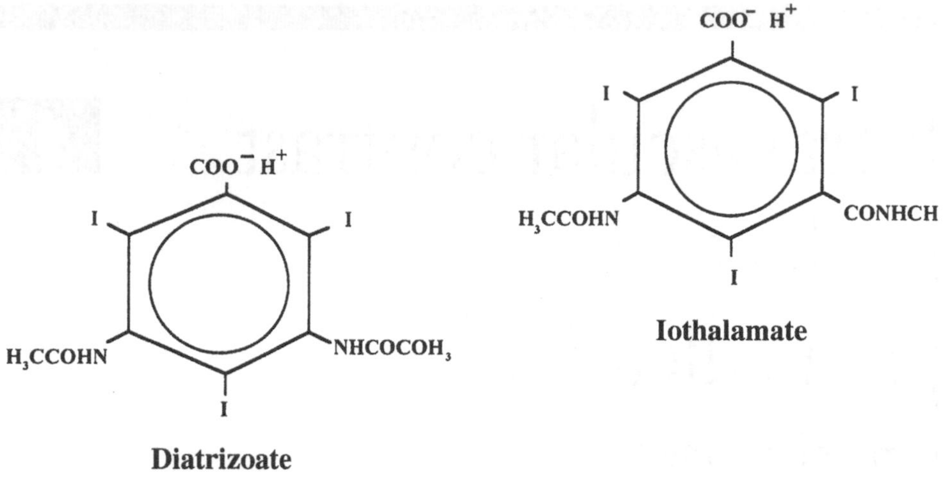

Figure 1.1 High-osmolality iodinated contrast media.

vs. dimers, grams of iodine, etc.). The most practical method of classification is according to osmolality (See Table 1.1).

High-osmolality contrast media

High-osmolality contrast media are ionic salts that dissociate into a cation and anion in solution. There are two basic types of high-osmolality ionic iodinated contrast media. The first is diatrizoate (Fig. 1.1), which was introduced in 1953, is contained in numerous products, and is the most widely used contrast medium in the world for urography, angiography and CT. The two side-chains improve the molecule's solubility and reduce protein binding, and therefore increase its ability to be filtered in the glomerulus. The second type of ionic iodinated contrast agent is iothalamate (Fig. 1.1). Iothalamate is exactly the same as diatrizoate, except that there is a substitution of one of the two nitrogen atoms on one of the organic side-chains by a carboxyl group. This led to better neural tolerance but was less well tolerated by the cardiovascular system. Diatrizoate is the primary agent utilized in most ionic contrast media (Renovist®, Hypaque®, Renografin®, Reno-M-Dip®). Only one manufacturer offers an iothalamate agent (Conray®).

Both iothalamate and diatrizoate are classified as salts, and therefore have to be manufactured in solution with a cation other than hydrogen. Most agents use sodium or meglumine or mixtures of sodium/meglumine for their cation. Meglumine is a 6-carbon sugar with a positive charge, and is better tolerated by the central nervous system and peripheral blood vessels than sodium. Pure sodium salts tend to cause more burning sensation at angiography and tend to result in more CNS toxicity or seizures. Therefore, whenever these agents are used in neurovascular imaging, pure meglumine salts are preferred.

Use in coronary angiography is unique in that one has to use a sodium concentration in the contrast media that is the same as the sodium concentration found in the body. Therefore, most cardiac angiography was performed with a combination of sodium/meglumine that resulted in a sodium concentration similar to the serum concentration of sodium. This concentration of sodium results in less disruption of the sodium–potassium pump at the cell membrane level of the heart. Hypaque-76® and Renografin-76® are examples of these agents. They have a sodium: meglumine ratio of 1:6.6. However, most practices, have switched to nonionic contrast media for cardiac angiography.

As mentioned earlier, because of the ionic nature of diatrizoate and iothalamate contrast media, these agents dissociate into a cation and an anion in solution. This results in two particles in solution for every particle administered. Because of this, these agents have a relatively high osmolality (1500–2100 mOsm/kg water) compared to serum (300 mOsm/kg water). It is felt that many of the side-effects of contrast media are caused entirely or mainly by their excessively high osmolality. These side-effects include vascular pain or burning, endothelial cell damage, disturbances of the blood–brain barrier, thrombosis and thrombophlebitis, bradycardia, and increases in pulmonary arterial pressure.

Lower-osmolality contrast media

In the course of the 1960s, it became increasingly clear that many of the side-effects of conventional intravenous contrast media were caused more by the high osmolality of the contrast medium than by the chemotoxicity of the agent. Torsten Almen, a radiologist from Sweden, developed the first lower-osmolality contrast medium metrizamide (Amipaque®). The osmolality of metrizamide was approximately 650 mOsm/kg. This agent was first introduced for myelograms. It was the first water-soluble agent that could be introduced into the subarachnoid space safely and did not have to be physically removed like Pantopaque®, but rather was absorbed by the body and excreted by the kidneys via glomerular filtration.

Lower-osmolality contrast media – monomers　The unique feature that Torsten Almen developed was the replacement of the ionic carboxyl group in position 1 by an organic side-chain. This not only made the new compound nonionic, but also reduced its osmolality in solution because it did not dissociate into two particles (anion and cation). This lowering of the osmolality resulted in less vascular pain, less disturbance of the blood–brain barrier, less bradycardia and less increase in pressure of the pulmonary arterial circulation.

Because metrizamide had some chemotoxicity problems, it was quickly replaced by the second generation of nonionic lower-osmolality contrast media, (namely iopamidol (Isovue®, Bracco), iohexol (Omnipaque®, Nycomed), ioversol (Optiray®, Mallinckrodt), iopromide (Ultravist®, Berlex) and ioxilan (Oxilan®, Cook) (Fig. 1.2). These five agents are all nonionic and are lower in osmolality than conventional ionic contrast media (Table 1.2). These newer agents were better tolerated than metrizamide. Because of this, metrizamide is no longer marketed in the USA.

Lower-osmolality contrast media – dimers　In addition it is possible to produce a low-osmolality contrast medium that is also ionic. This is done by combining a

(a)

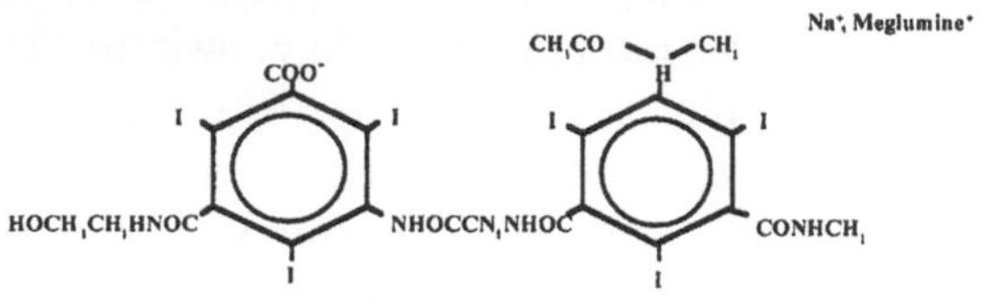

– ioxaglate (Hexabrix)

(b)

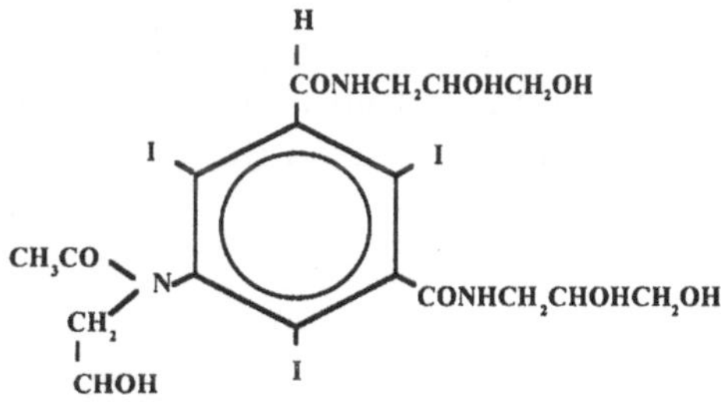

– iohexol (Omnipaque)

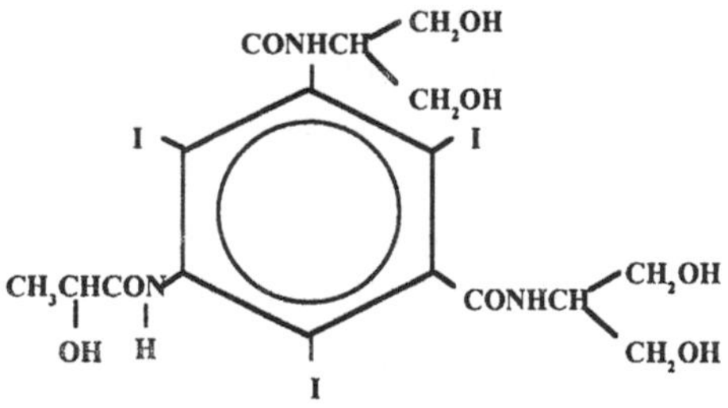

– iopamidol (Isovue)

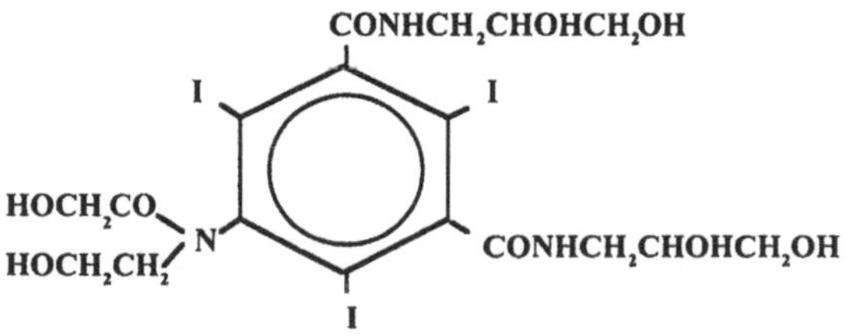

– ioversol (Optiray)

(c)

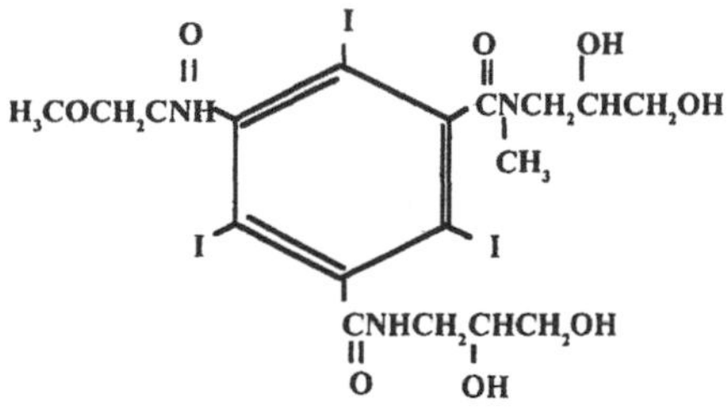

– iopromide (Ultravist)

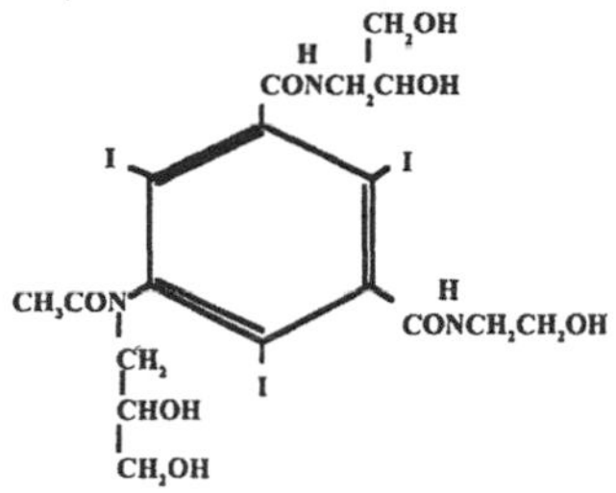

– ioxilan (Oxilan)

(d)

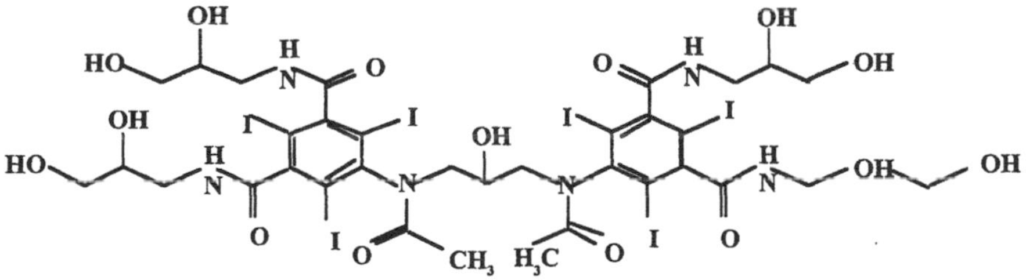

– iodixanol (Visipaque)

Figure 1.2 Low-osmolality iodinated contrast media: (a) ionic dimer; (b) and (c) non-ionic monomers; and (d) nonionic dimers.

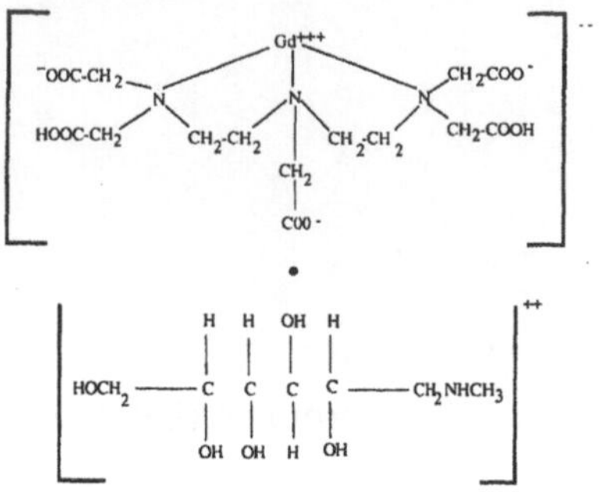

Gd-DTPA (Magnevist)

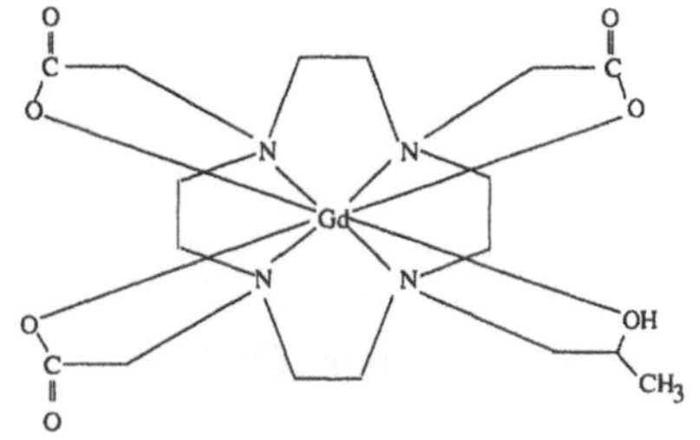

Gd-HP-DO3A (ProHance)

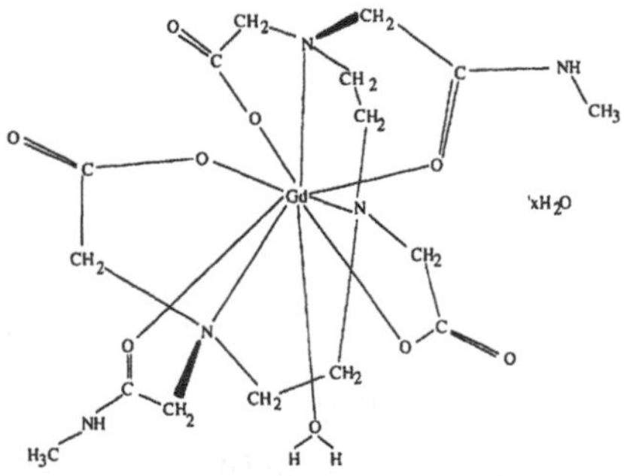

Gd-DTPA-GMA (Omniscan)

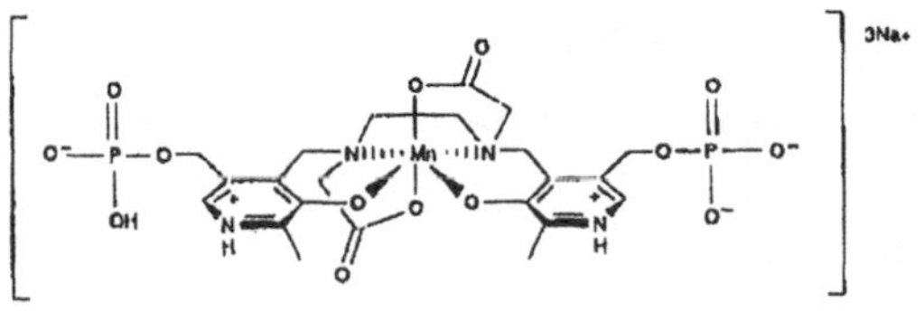

Mangafodipir trisodium (Teslascan)
'Manganese + fodipir'

Figure 1.3   MRI contrast agents.

nonionic tri-iodinated benzene ring with an ionic tri-iodinated benzene ring (Fig. 1.2). This results in a dimer with a total of six iodine atoms per molecule. However, when this dimer is injected intravenously, it quickly dissociates into the large dimer anion and a positively charged cation (meglumine or sodium). The only available ionic dimer is ioxaglate (Hexabrix®). The osmolality of ioxaglate is essentially the same as that of nonionic monomers such as iopamidol, iohexol and ioversol (Table 1.2).

Table 1.1 Classification of iodinated and MRI contrast media

Classification of iodinated contrast media	
High-osmolality	
Ionic (monomers)	Iothalamate (Conray)
	Diatrizoate (Renovist, Hypaque, Renografin)
Low-osmolality	
Ionic (dimer)	Ioxaglate (Hexabrix)
Nonionic (monomer)	Iohexol (Omnipaque)
	Iopamidol (Isovue)
	Ioversol (Optiray)
	Iopromide (Ultravist)
	Ioxilan (Oxilan)
Nonionic (dimer)	Iodixanol (Visipaque)
Classification of MRI contrast media	
Gadolinium ionic	
Gd-DTPA	Magnevist (Berlex)
Gadolinium nonionic	
Gd-HP-DO3A Gadoteridol	ProHance (Bracco)
Gd-DTPA-GMA Gadodiamide	Omniscan (Nycomed Amersham)
Organ specific	
Ferrous oxide	Feridex (Berlex)
Mangafodipir trisodium (manganese + fodipir)	Teslascan (Nycomed Amersham)

A nonionic dimer has also been introduced. This agent is iodixanol (Visapaque), which is made by combining two nonionic monomers. This results in a dimer with a total of six iodine atoms per molecule. When this dimer is injected, it stays in solution as one particle, and therefore has the lowest osmolality of all iodinated contrast agents (290 mOsm/kg water). However, it has a higher viscosity of 11 cP at 37°C.

Formulations

Intravascular X-ray contrast media are usually available as ready-to-inject solutions. Nonionic contrast media and highly concentrated forms of contrast media (Angiovist® and Renografin-76® and Hypaque-90®) are more viscous, and usually require heating to body temperature prior to intravenous or intra-arterial injection.

Because of the various components in these contrast agents, attention must be paid to the following properties: (a) the type and amount (weight/volume concentration) of the active ingredient, (b) where applicable, the type and mixture of salts, and (c) the iodine concentration in mg/mL. The actual concentration of the contrast agent chemical in water is of less relevance clinically than the iodine

Table 1.2 Diagnostic imaging intravascular contrast agents

Product structure	Chemical ionic status	Anion	Cation	Iodine (mg/mL)	Viscosity 37°C (cP)	Osmolality (mOsm/kg water)
High-osmolality iodinated contrast media						
Renovue®-DIP (Bracco)	Ionic	Iodamine	Meglumine	c.111	1.8	433
Reno-M-DIP® (Bracco)	Ionic	Diatrizoate	Meglumine	141	1.4	644
Reno-M-60® (Bracco)	Ionic	Diatrizoate	Meglumine	282	4.0	1404
Renografin®-60 (Bracco)	Ionic	Diatrizoate	Meglumine 52 sodium 8	292	4.0	1450
Renografin®-76 (Bracco)	Ionic	Diatrizoate	Meglumine 66 sodium 10	370	8.4	1940
Conray® 30 (Mallinckrodt)	Ionic	Iothalamate	Meglumine	141	c.1.5	c.600
Conray® 43 (Mallinckrodt)	Ionic	Iothalamate	Meglumine	202	c.2	c.1000
Conray® 60 (Mallinckrodt)	Ionic	Iothalamate	Meglumine	282	4	1400
Conray® 400 (Mallinckrodt)	Ionic	Iothalamate	Sodium	400	4.5	2300
Hypaque® Meglumine 30% (Nycomed)	Ionic	Diatrizoate	Meglumine	141	1.43	633
Hypaque® (Nycomed)	Ionic	Diatrizoate	Meglumine	370	4.5	1800
Hypaque® Meglumine 60% (Nycomed)	Ionic	Diatrizoate	Meglumine	282	4.1	1415
Hypaque® 76 Meglumine 6% (Nycomed)	Ionic	Diatrizoate	Meglumine 66 sodium 10	282	4.1	1415
Urovist® Meglumine DIU/CT (Berlex)	Ionic	Diatrizoate	Meglumine	141	1.4	640
Angiovist® 282 (Berlex)	Ionic	Diatrizoate	Meglumine	282	4.1	1400
Angiovist® 370 (Berlex)	Ionic	Diatrizoate	Meglumine 66 sodium 10	370	8.4	2100
Low-osmolality iodinated contrast media						
Optiray® 160 (Mallinckrodt)	Nonionic monomer (ioversol)	–	–	160	1.9	355
Optiray® 240 (Mallinckrodt)	Nonionic monomer (ioversol)	–	–	240	3.0	502
Optiray® 320 (Mallinckrodt)	Nonionic monomer (ioversol)	–	–	320	5.8	702
Isovue®-200 (Bracco) 40.8%)	Nonionic monomer (iopamidol)	–	–	200	2.0	413
Isovue®-300 (Bracco)	Nonionic monomer (iopamidol)	–	–	300	6.8	616

Table 1.2 *continued*

Product structure	Chemical ionic status	Anion	Cation	Iodine (mg/mL)	Viscosity 37°C (cP)	Osmolality (mOsm/ kg water)
Iosvue® 370	Nonionic monomer	–	–	370	10	774
Omnipaque® 240 (Nycomed)	Nonionic monomer (iohexol)	–	–	240	3.4	520
Omnipaque® 300 (Nycomed)	Nonionic monomer (iohexol)	–	–	300	7.5	709
Ultravist® 150 (Berlex)	Nonionic monomer (iopromide)	–	–	150	1.8	300
Ultravist® 240 (Berlex)	Nonionic monomer (iopromide)	–	–	240	2.8	483
Ultravist® 300 (Berlex)	Nonionic monomer (iopromide)	–	–	300	4.9	607
Ultravist® 370 (Berlex)	Nonionic monomer (iopromide)	–	–	370	10.0	774
Oxilan® 300 (Cook)	Nonionic monomer (oxilan)	–	–	300	5.1	585
Oxilan® 350 (Cook)	Nonionic monomer (oxilan)	–	–	350	8.1	695
Visipaque® 270 (Nycomed)	Nonionic dimer (iodixanol)	–	–	270	6.3	290
Visipaque® 320 (Nycomed)	Nonionic dimer (iodixanol)	–	–	320	11.8	290
Hexabrix® (Mallinckrodt)	Ionic dimer (ioxaglate)	Ioxaglate	Na (19.6%) Meglumine (39.3%)	320	4.7	600
MR contrast media						
Magnevist® (Berlex)	Ionic	Gd-DTPA	Meglumine	–	4.9	1940
ProHance® (Bracco)	Nonionic Gd-HP-D03A (Gadoteridol)	–	–	–	2.0	630
Omniscan® (Nycomed)	Nonionic Gd-DTPA-GMA (Gadodiamide)	–	–	–	2.0	789
Feridex® (Berlex)	Ferrous oxide Mannitol Dextran	–	–	–	–	340
Teslascan® (Nycomed)	Mangafodipir trisodium (manganese + fodipir)	(MnDPDP)	Na+	–	0.8	298

concentration in mg/mL. Because iodine is the only portion of these agents that contributes to opacification, it becomes the main ingredient that requires appropriate attention. Various examinations require low iodine concentration, such as cystography of the bladder. Other agents require high concentrations of iodine, such as angiography of small blood vessels in the head or coronary arteries. In addition, it is believed that some adverse events associated with these agents may be directly related to the total number of grams of iodine given to the patient.

Therefore, one should be fully aware of the relative number of grams of iodine in the contrast medium being administered (Table 1.2).

In addition to the contrast medium, the finished preparations also contain pharmacologically relevant adjuvants. $CaNa_2EDTA$ is one of these agents, and is virtually inactive at the concentrations and dosages used. It is employed as a stabilizer in order to prevent the release of iodide from the organic bond caused by heavy metal catalysis. Buffers such as TRIS and carbonate buffers are often added to stabilize the pH during storage.

Physiology

Renal clearance

Because of very minimal protein binding and their small molecular size, iodinated contrast media are almost totally eliminated by the kidneys via glomerular filtration. In normal individuals, 98 per cent is eliminated by glomerular filtration, and less than 2 per cent is excreted by liver, bowel and salivary glands. The half-life of contrast media before being eliminated into the bladder is approximately 30 min in healthy individuals and 1–2 h in elderly patients. Immediately after injection of intravenous iodinated contrast media, there is equilibration between the interstitial fluid (third space) and the intravascular fluid space. Because of this equilibration, clearance from the body follows an exponential rate. Virtually all of the intravenous iodinated contrast medium should be eliminated by 24 h after the examination. In fact, if a pyelogram is noted on an abdominal CT or on a plain film of the abdomen 24 h after the administration of IV contrast, this is considered abnormal and a sign of impaired clearance, most often due to impaired renal function.

Renal blood flow

Because of the high osmolality of conventional ionic contrast media, there is a biphasic change in renal blood flow following the administration of iodinated contrast medium. Initially, there is a transient increase (approximately 1 min) in renal blood flow, followed by an extended period of decreased blood flow (up to several hours). The lower-osmolality nonionic contrast media have less effect on renal blood flow.

Renal function

Contrast-induced injury to the kidneys can occur, and it appears to result from a combination of factors, including decreased blood flow, glomerular cellular injury or tubular cellular injury. This contrast-induced injury to the kidney does not appear to be dose related at lower doses (less than 30g of iodine). However, it may be dose related at higher doses (over 50g of iodine).

Patients with insulin-dependent diabetes and renal insufficiency (serum Cr > 1.5 mg/dL) are at a very high risk for contrast nephropathy. Diabetes alone or mild renal insufficiency alone appear to be minor risk factors. Repeated doses of contrast media on consecutive days and dehydration also appear to be major risk factors. Although lower-osmolality agents may result in less nephrotoxicity in patients with impaired renal function, no definite advantage has been seen with lower-osmolality contrast media in other patients. Adequate hydration has been shown to reduce the likelihood of contrast nephropathy and dehydration appears to be one of the most important factors in patients who have developed contrast nephropathy. This is particularly true for patients with any renal insufficiency.

Cardiac responses

Iodinated contrast media can produce cardiovascular responses that may result from direct action on the myocardium, pulmonary or peripheral vasculature, or may be mediated by the central or autonomic nervous systems. Specific cardiac actions are most often seen during coronary arterial injection, which causes acute depression of myocardial contractility followed by bradycardia. Coronary arteriography can also be associated with disturbances in conduction velocity and cardiac arrhythmias. These effects appear to be more pronounced with higher-osmolality contrast media.

Peripheral vasculature

Intravenous and intra-arterial injections of contrast media produce a peripheral vasodilatation mediated by the direct effect of the higher osmolality of the contrast media on the vasculature. This results in a decrease in peripheral vascular resistance, a reflex fall in blood pressure, an increase in cardiac output and an increase in blood volume. This peripheral vasodilatation is often perceived by the patient to be a sensation of heat and pain, which is primarily a function of the osmolality. These findings are less pronounced with the newer lower-osmolality contrast media.

Pulmonary responses

The pulmonary responses to injection of contrast media into the pulmonary artery are an elevated pulmonary arterial pressure and a reduced mean aortic pressure. It is believed that these high-osmolality solutions withdraw water from the erythrocytes, making them more rigid and temporarily increasing pulmonary vascular resistance, leading to increased pulmonary arterial pressure.

In addition, iodinated contrast media can also destabilize mast-cell membranes. Because a large proportion of mast cells within the body reside in the lung, iodinated contrast media can result in the release of histamine from the mast cells and cause hives, bronchospasm, coughing, respiratory arrest, laryngeal edema, or peripheral vasodilatation and shock. This destabilization of mast cells appears to be related to the higher osmolality, and is less pronounced with lower-osmolality contrast media.

Rarely, pulmonary edema can occur in response to large doses of contrast media, and it appears to increase with the dose and rate of injection, but does not seem to be related to the osmolality.

Neurovascular responses

The immediate effects of intracarotid injections of hyperosmolal contrast media can be bradycardia and hypotension, caused by the direct action on the vagal brain centers and on receptors in the carotid body. Repeated injections of hyperosmolal contrast media appear to lower the seizure threshold, as a result of the chemotoxic action of contrast media on exposed neurons. This is believed to occur most commonly when the blood–brain barrier has been penetrated by the contrast media, which can be seen in repeated injections of hyperosmolal contrast media, or in pathologic conditions where the blood–brain barrier is interrupted. Meglumine salts of high-osmolality contrast media appear to have less deleterious effects than sodium salts. However, lower-osmolality contrast media are superior in terms of reduced toxicity in animal experiments. In clinical studies, the newer lower-osmolality contrast media are preferable in terms of their milder production of EEG changes, bradycardia and hypotension. In addition, because the external carotid artery is opacified during common carotid artery injections, there is much less vascular pain in the face and neck when lower-osmolality contrast media are used.

Endothelial effects

Contrast media have a local irritant effect on the vascular endothelium, which appears to be the result of a combination of chemotoxicity and hypertonicity. This is most important in phlebography of the lower extremity due to prolonged periods of exposure to the highly concentrated media. It is believed that venous thrombosis is an occasional serious consequence of this interaction when contrast medium injures endothelial cells and begins the process of platelet aggregation and clot formation. This endothelial toxicity factor also appears to play an important role in the initiation of anaphylactoid reactions. Low-osmolality contrast media appear to result in less endothelial cell damage because their tonicity is closer to that of blood.

Clotting mechanisms

All iodinated contrast media appear to inhibit the clotting mechanism within the body. This appears to be directly related to the higher osmolality of the contrast media. The relative inhibition of coagulation by intravenous contrast media appears to be due to a combination of inhibition of platelet aggregation and limitation of the clotting cascade mechanism. There is more clotting inhibition with the high-osmolality contrast media than there is with the lower-osmolality contrast media. Although meticulous technique should be used at all times during flushing of catheters in angiography, one should be cognizant of the fact that lower-osmolality contrast media retard clotting less when blood and contrast media mix in these catheters. This is extremely important during coronary or cerebral angiography.

Adverse reactions to iodinated contrast media

The adverse effects of intravenous iodinated contrast media can be divided into two categories, namely adverse physiologic effects (predictable) and adverse reactions (unpredictable and idiosyncratic). We have discussed the many adverse physiologic effects that are predictable, such as the sensation of heat and pain following the intravenous or intra-arterial injection of contrast media. In addition, an alteration in heart rate and a decrease in cardiac contractility in response to intracardiac injections are other predictable adverse physiologic effects. The second group of adverse reactions are less predictable, occur uncommonly, and appear to be due to a number of possible mechanisms, including histamine release (hives, asthma, laryngeal edema), CNS toxicity (seizures, rigors, vasovagal) and cardiac toxicity (cardiac arrest, arrhythmias, hypotension/cardiovascular collapse). The overall incidences of some adverse physiologic effects and reactions are listed in Table 1.3.

Table 1.3 Incidence of adverse reactions[a] to contrast media

	Iodinated contrast media	
High-osmolality contrast media (%)	Adverse reactions	Lower-osmolality contrast media (%)
6.0	Nausea and vomiting	1.0
3.0	Urticaria	0.5
2.6	Hoarseness, sneezing, cough, dyspnea or facial edema	0.5
0.1	Drop in blood pressure	0.01
	MRI contrast media[b]	
Contrast media	Adverse reactions	Incidence (%)
Gadolinium chelates	Mild (nausea and/or vomiting)	2.0
	Moderate	0.1
	Severe	0.01
Ferrous oxide	Aching muscles	8.0
	Others (including allergic-like reactions)	3.0
Manganese fodipir	Injection site discomfort	67.0
	Nausea and/or vomiting	14.0
	Headache	5.0
	Others	<1.0

[a]Adapted from Katayama et al.
[b]Mayo experience.

Lower-osmolality vs. high-osmolality contrast media

Early in the 1980s, lower-osmolality contrast media were introduced for intravascular use in diagnostic radiology imaging. These agents have been found to have a lower incidence of mild, moderate and severe reactions. Since 1990, the American College of Radiology (ACR) and others have studied the potential benefits of lower-osmolality contrast media vs. high-osmolality contrast media. A general set of potential guidelines reflecting our experience as well as that of others is included at the end of this section for the reader's information (Box 1.1).

MRI contrast media

Intravenous contrast agents in magnetic resonance imaging (MRI) are unique in that their effect is to change the T-1 and T-2 relaxation times of various tissues. There are a number of ways of achieving changes in T-1 and T-2 relaxation times of tissues. However, most efforts have concentrated on intravenous paramagnetic or ferromagnetic substances.

The mechanism whereby paramagnetic agents provide contrast differs from the way in which radiographic contrast media work. X-ray contrast media are observed directly on radiographic images because of their ability to absorb X-rays. However, the paramagnetic MRI contrast agents operate in an indirect manner by altering the local magnetic environment of tissues. Chemicals that have unpaired electrons (e.g. transition or lanthanide metal ions, organic free radicals) are the most effective paramagnetic contrast enhancers. This is so because the magnetic moments of unpaired electrons are 657 times larger than the magnetic moments of unpaired protons or neutrons. Thus paramagnetic substances have a permanent magnetism due to their spin moment caused by an unpaired electron. In the absence of external magnetic fields, the magnetic moments of paramagnetic substances are randomly aligned. However, with the application of a strong external magnetic field, the magnetic moments align with the field and generate strong local magnetic fields that shorten both T-1 and T-2 relaxation times of neighboring protons. When paramagnetic ions are added to water, the relaxation process of water molecules is more enhanced in the vicinity of these paramagnetic centers.

Although these transition and lanthanide inorganic cations are powerful proton relaxers, the free metal ions are extremely toxic for human use. Because of the toxicity of these free metal ions, chelated metal complexes have been proposed and developed for MRI. Chelating agents such as EDTA and diethylenetriaminepentaacetic acid (DTPA) utilize strong ligand bonds to bind to these toxic metal ions. These chelating complexes protect the free metal ions from combining with circulating proteins or cellular membranes. The chelating complex of DTPA with gadolinium resulted in the first safe intravenous MRI contrast agent, known as gadolinium-DTPA (Magnevist®). Recently, two new gadolinium chelating complexes have been released

BOX 1.1 GUIDELINES ON THE APPROPRIATE USE OF IODINATED CONTRAST MEDIA

1 Conventional high-osmolality contrast media have been used for decades and continue to be safe and effective contrast media for intravascular use.

2 Pretreatment of patients with two or three doses of steroids prior to contrast administration can reduce the incidence of subsequent contrast reactions. Steroid pretreatment can also reduce the incidence of reactions in individuals who have experienced a previous severe contrast adverse reaction.

3 In all patients, especially those with a previous contrast reaction, consideration should be given to the need to administer contrast media. Acceptable alternative imaging procedures that can be performed without intravascular contrast media should be sought. If contrast medium is to be used, the smallest amount that will provide a diagnostic study should be utilized.

4 High standards should be maintained in screening patients for risk factors prior to administration of intravenous contrast media. Prompt recognition and proper treatment of contrast reactions should continue to be a top priority in all radiology departments.

5 Based on the available data at this time, each radiologist should make his or her own decision about the type of contrast medium to be used for each patient. Situations that might alert the radiologist to consider using lower-osmolality contrast media are:
   - patients with a previous significant adverse reaction to contrast media or a history of allergies or asthma;
   - patients with cardiac dysfunction, including a history of arrhythmias, angina pectoris, recent myocardial infarction, pulmonary hypertension or congestive heart failure;
   - patients with generalized debilitation. This would include patients who are hemodynamically unstable, or hospitalized patients with multiple medical problems. Elderly patients who may not tolerate a mild or moderate contrast reaction may fall into this category;
   - patients undergoing potentially painful examinations such as peripheral angiography, carotid angiography and lower limb phlebography;
   - patients undergoing examinations such as digital angiography or bolus CT examinations, where inadvertent motion must be minimized in order to optimize image quality;
   - patients who are overly anxious about contrast administration.

6 Although written informed consent has been advocated by some authors, it has been concluded that the available data concerning this issue are incomplete. Each radiologist should check with hospital bylaws as well as local and state laws regarding this issue.

BOX 1.1 *continued*

7 Impaired renal function continues to be a risk factor for contrast nephropathy. This is especially true in diabetic patients. Patients with impaired renal function may experience less renal injury from lower-osmolality contrast media. Attention should be given to providing adequate hydration prior to the exam and adequate fluid intake after it.

8 Efforts should continue to bring down the price of lower-osmolality contrast media at the local and national level. Competitive pricing techniques should continue to be used.

9 A uniform method should be established for recording the type and amount of contrast medium used and any adverse effects at each locale. This information could be recorded on the radiology examination report. This data will facilitate quality assurance and contribute to our understanding of contrast media and their effects at each locale.

Note: These are only potential guidelines. Various practices may differ, and we realize that these guidelines cannot apply to all practice situations.

for intravenous use, Gd-HP-DO3A (ProHance®) and Gd-DTPA-BMA (Omniscan®) (Table 1.2 and Fig. 1.3).

A major concern about the intravenous use of metal chelates is the potential for *in-vivo* dissociation of the complexes, which would release toxic free metal ions. This may be important in patients with impaired renal function who may have prolonged retention of these complexes. Therefore, a preparation of metal complexes with a high stability constant is required.

The gadolinium chelates that are utilized in MRI in current practice carry a very small risk of contrast reactions. Although anecdotal reports of life-threatening reactions to these agents have been made, the precise incidence of severe life-threatening reactions is uncertain. However, it is generally believed that severe life-threatening reactions to gadolinium most probably occur in 1:100 000 patients (compared to ionic, iodinated agents → 1:1000 and nonionic, iodinated agents → 1:6000).

At the present time there does not appear to be any significant difference in the safety and efficacy of the three gadolinium-based MRI agents. Most gadolinium-based MRI agents are approved for 'triple' dosing and rapid injection.

An iron-based, liver-specific contrast medium has recently been approved by the FDA (Feridex®, Berlex). This agent is picked up by the reticulo-endothelial (RE) cells of the liver. This new agent decreases the signal intensity of normal liver tissue on T-2 weighted images, and therefore makes high-signal tumors more conspicuous.

Another liver-specific MRI contrast agent has also been recently introduced. This agent is mangafodipir, which is formed as a complex between a chelating agent (fodipir) and a paramagnetic metal ion, manganese. Mangafodipir shortens the T-1 relaxation time of targeted tissues such as the liver, leading to an increase in signal intensity.

Adverse reactions to MRI contrast media

Adverse reactions to gadolinium-based contrast media for MRI are very rare. However, they still can occur. Headaches are the most common adverse effects, occurring in 3 per cent of patients. Nausea or vomiting is the next most common adverse effect and occurs in 1–2 per cent of patients. Routinely keeping patients NPO (nothing by mouth) for 6–12 h prior to the MRI study may help to reduce the risk of vomiting in the scanner.

Anaphylactoid reactions to gadolinium-based contrast media are rare (<1 per cent). However, they can and do occur. Therefore, all MRI sites that administer gadolinium-based contrast media should be prepared to treat anaphylactoid reactions. Death due to gadolinium contrast agents has been reported. Active bronchospasm or severe chronic obstructive pulmonary disease (COPD) with a bronchospastic component were present in these fatal cases. Therefore, gadolinium should be given cautiously or not at all to patients with active bronchospasm.

Anaphylactoid reactions can occur (0.5 per cent) with liver-specific, iron-based, MRI contrast agents (Feridex®, Berlex). These ferumoxides are colloids of iron oxide with dextran. Muscle or back pain can occur in up to 8 per cent of patients receiving these iron-based, liver MRI agents. In 2.5 per cent of these patients the pain is severe enough to result in the interruption or cessation of the infusion.

Adverse reactions can also occur with manganese fodipir agents. The most common adverse event is discomfort at the injection site (67 per cent) which can be minimized by injecting slowly over 2–3 min. Nausea or vomiting may occur in up to 14 per cent of patients, and keeping patients NPO prior to the MRI study may help. Serious life-threatening reactions can occur, but appear to be rare (0.3 per cent).

Etiology of adverse (idiosyncratic) reactions

There has always been confusion with regard to naming the idiosyncratic reactions to iodinated contrast material. They have been referred to by an assortment of terms, including allergic, idiosyncratic and anaphylactoid. The confusion stems from the fact that the reactions show similarities to allergic reactions, but they do not appear to fit some of the criteria for classic allergy. The outward manifestations of contrast reactions (urticaria, bronchospasm, laryngeal edema and cardiovascular collapse) are all consistent with allergic reactions, but other features of allergic reactions (such as circulating IgE antibodies) are not so clearly associated with reactions to iodinated contrast material.

Therefore, the exact etiology and nature of idiosyncratic or anaphylactoid reactions following the administration of intravascular contrast media are not fully understood. There are three possible etiologies, namely histamine release, complement activation and allergic reaction.

Histamine is stored and released by mast cells or basophils when degranulation occurs within the cells. There is both *in-vitro* and *in-vivo* evidence to substantiate the claim that histamine is released from basophils in the presence of iodinated contrast material. Nonionic, lower-osmolality agents do not seem to have the same histamine-releasing capability as ionic high-osmolality agents, at least *in vitro*. Histamine release appears to be greater during reactions to contrast material, and *in-vitro* challenges of reactor leukocytes appear to support this conclusion. A primary question that remains unanswered is whether histamine release plays a significant role in the reactions, or whether it is little more than a marker.

There is abundant *in-vitro* and *in-vivo* evidence that the complement system may be activated during contrast administration. Activation of the complement system not only results in the release of histamine, but also releases much more powerful agents such as kallikreins and leukokinins. The exact manner in which contrast media activate the complement system is not understood, nor is it understood why some individuals activate the complement system more than others, resulting in these rare anaphylactoid reactions. However, it is known that complement activation can be produced by ionic, nonionic, hypertonic and isotonic agents. Iodine does not appear to be a requirement, but the benzene-ring structure seems to be important. Early work has shown that there is a fall in complement factors in both normal patients and patients who have contrast reactions. However, patients with contrast reactions appear to show a greater sensitivity, at least *in vitro*, to contrast-induced complement activation.

Classic allergy requires a sensitizing exposure, yet many patients have reactions to contrast material at their initial exposure. In addition, patients who have had a contrast reaction may have no reaction on the next exposure. Moreover, classic allergy requires mediation through immune globulins but, in general, circulating antibodies to contrast material have not been identified. Unknown cofactors such as circulating haptens may play a role.

In summary, the exact etiology of anaphylaxis-like reactions due to intravenous iodinated contrast material is not well understood. Many of these reactions appear to be mediated by potent vasodilators such as histamines, kallikreins and leukokinins, which are probably released after some initiation of the complement cascade systems. Why and how this complement system is activated in some individuals and not in others is not yet understood.

Drug interaction

Renal toxicity has been reported in a few patients with liver dysfunction who were given a cholecystographic agent followed by intravascular iodinated contrast media. No medications should be mixed with iodinated contrast media.

Because glomerular filtration may be transiently impaired after exposure to contrast media, caution should be exercised in utilizing nephrotoxic drugs or drugs that need to be eliminated by the kidney. Glucophage® (metformin) is an oral diabetic agent that is cleared by the kidney. Accumulation of excessive amounts of Glucophage® may result in the depletion of available glucose, and could result in lactic acidosis. It is therefore recommended that Glucophage® be discontinued for 48 h after intravascular iodinated contrast media in order to prevent the excessive accumulation of Glucophage® and the potential for lactic acidosis.

Premedication

The best treatment for contrast reactions is *prevention*. Adequate screening of patients may identify individual patients who should not receive iodinated contrast media for various reasons (e.g. renal insufficiency, previous life-threatening reaction, active bronchospasm or asthma, hypotension or shock from an underlying illness, etc.).

In addition, several researchers have shown that premedication with corticosteriods prior to contrast administration will decrease the incidence of moderate and severe reactions. There are two recommended protocols for pretreatment of patients who are 'at risk' and who require contrast media. These pretreatment protocols are as follows:

1 Lasser approach:
   - 32 mg of Medrol® (methylprednisolone) p.o. 12 h and 2 h prior to IV administration of contrast medium.

2 Greenberger regimen:
   - prednisone – 50 mg p.o. 13 h, 7 h, and 1 h prior to the exam;
   - Benadryl® (diphenhydramine) – 50 mg p.o. 1 h prior to the exam;
   - ephedrine – 25 mg p.o. 1 h prior to the exam (contraindicated in patients with heart disease).

These pretreatment regimens have been shown to lower the incidence of subsequent contrast reactions compared to nontreated individuals. However, pretreatment with steroids will not prevent all contrast reactions, and adequate personnel, equipment and medication should be on hand for treatment of any subsequent reactions in these patients.

References

General
Katzberg RW (ed). *The contrast media manual.* Baltimore, MD: Williams and Wilkins, 1992.

Parvez Z (ed). *Contrast media: biologic effects and clinical application. Volumes I, II, III.* Boca Raton, FL: CRC Press, 1987.

Skucas J (ed). *Radiographic contrast agents*, 2nd edn. Rockville, MD: Aspen Publishers, 1989.

Swanson DP, Shetty PC, Kastan DJ, Rollins N. Angiographic contrast media. In: Swanson DP, Chilton HM, Thrall JH, eds. *Pharmaceuticals in medical imaging.* New York: Macmillan, 1990; 13–39.

Lower-osmolality contrast medium
Bettmann MA. Ionic versus nonionic contrast agents for intravenous use: are all the answers in? *Radiology* 1990; **175**: 616–18.

Katayama H, Yamaguchi K, Kozuka T, Takashima T, Seez P, Matsuura K. Adverse reactions to ionic and nonionic contrast media: a report from the Japanese Committee on the Safety of Contrast Media. *Radiology* 1990; **175**: 621–8.

Palmer FJ. The Royal Australasian College of Radiology survey of intravenous contrast media reactions: final report. *Australasian Radiology* 1988; **32**: 426–8.

Wolf GL, Arenson RL, Cross AP. A prospective trial of ionic vs nonionic contrast agents in routine clinical practice: comparison of adverse effects. *American Journal of Roentgenology* 1989; **152**: 939–44.

Nephrotoxicity
Lautin EM, Freeman NJ, Schoenfeld AH *et al.* Radiocontrast-associated renal dysfunction: incidence and risk factors. *American Journal of Roentgenology* 1991; **157**: 49–58.

Schwab SJ, Hlatky MA, Peiper KS *et al.* Contrast nephrotoxicity: a randomized controlled trial of a nonionic and an ionic radiographic contrast agent. *New England Journal of Medicine* 1989; **320**: 149–53.

Taliercio CP, Vlietstra RE, Ilstrup DM *et al.* A randomized comparison of the nephrotoxicity of iopamidol and diatrizoate in high-risk patients undergoing cardiac angiography. *Journal of the American College of Cardiology* 1991; **17**: 384–90.

MRI contrast media
Carr JJ. Magnetic resonance contrast agents for neuroimaging. Safety issues. *Neuroimaging Clinics of North America* 1994; **4**: 43–54.

Federle MP, Chezmar JL, Rubin MD *et al.* The efficacy and safety of mangafodipir trisodium (MnDPDP) injection for hepatic MRI in adults. Part 1. Early imaging (in press).

Goldstein HA, Kashaniau FK, Blumetti RF, Lolyoak WL, Hugo FP, Blumenfield DM. Safety assessment of gadopentate dimeglumine in US clinical trials. *Radiology* 1990; **174**: 17–23.

Murphy KJ, Brunberg JA, Cohan RH. Adverse reactions to gadolinium contrast media: a review of 36 cases. *American Journal of Roentgenology* 1996; **167**: 847–9.

Niendorf HP, Haustein J, Cornelius I, Alhassan A, Clauss W. Safety of gadolinium-DTPA: extended clinical experience. *Magnetic Resonance in Medicine* 1991; **22**: 222–8.

Salonen OLM. Case of anaphylaxis and four cases of allergic reaction following Gd-DTPA administration. *Journal of Computer-Assisted Tomography* 1990; **14**: 912–13.

2 Presentation and early recognition of contrast reactions*

Karl N. Krecke

Sooner or later, nearly every practising radiologist will encounter a patient with a severe reaction to contrast material.[1] The relatively low incidence but high risk to the patient requires prompt recognition and focused treatment by the radiologist and allied personnel.

Minor reactions, consisting mainly of cutaneous reactions of urticaria, local erythema or nasal congestion, occur in approximately one in 20 to 50 injections of high-osmolar contrast material (HOCM).[2,3] Severe reactions occur less commonly, in approximately one in 1000 injections, and rapid diagnosis and treatment are necessary to arrest progression and prevent death. While moderate to severe reactions are unanticipated, the abrupt, dramatic presentation and context of contrast-material administration make the diagnosis readily apparent. This situation is a complication of medical care, and the physician and staff must at all times be prepared to diagnose and treat. Rapid, considered action is paramount to the patient's recovery, and possibly to his or her survival.

True anaphylaxis is an exaggerated allergic reaction to a foreign substance. By strict criteria, it requires antigen–antibody interaction with mast cells and basophils that respond with the release of histamine and other vasoactive substances. Histamine, bradykinins and leukotrienes are well-accepted mediators of anaphylaxis, and vasoactive prostaglandins and complement factors are considered to be likely mediators of systemic reactions. Ionic contrast media have been reported to liberate or activate all of these, with the exception of the leukotrienes. Consequently, administration of contrast media can result in release or activation of identical mediators, causing identical end organ responses in an anaphylaxis-like, or anaphylactoid, syndrome.[4] The highest concentrations of mast cells are associated with blood vessels, skin, respiratory tract and gastrointestinal tract (Table 2.1).[5]

*From King BF Jr, Krecke KN, Prescott SL (Course Directors): *Advanced Radiology Life Support*™ (*ARLS*). © 1998, reproduced with permission of the Mayo Foundation.

Table 2.1 Findings in anaphylactoid syndromes

Skin	Pruritus, urticaria, angioedema, erythema
Eyes	Pruritus, conjunctival congestion
Nose	Sneezing, congestion, rhinorrhea
Mouth	Pruritus, edema
Upper airway	Hoarseness, stridor, laryngeal edema
Lower airway	Dyspnea, tachypnea, wheezing, rales, bronchospasm, pulmonary edema
Cardiovascular	Hypotension, tachycardia, arrhythmia
Gastrointestinal	Abdominal pain, cramping, diarrhea, nausea, vomiting

Simple inspection of the patient, palpation of the pulse, and auscultation of the neck and chest provide enough information to allow one to begin therapy. The severity and progression of signs and symptoms will determine specific choices of therapy and the need for additional emergency support.

The patient's position and demeanor will indicate the urgency of the situation and separate the differential diagnoses into manageable groups. *The uncomfortable, but calm, patient* is usually experiencing a cutaneous reaction which may or may not require treatment. The patient who is *anxious and agitated*, and often sitting up on the table, is most often suffering from respiratory compromise, most commonly laryngeal edema or bronchospasm. These are patients who very much need your attention. Patients suffering panic attacks may also manifest with symptoms of shortness of breath, palpitations and agitation. Less common reactions seen in this group of patients include pulmonary edema, hypoglycemia, hypertensive reactions and rigors. The *subdued or unresponsive* patient is generally suffering from cardiovascular decline, due to either vasovagal reaction or diffuse vasodilation and hypotension.

Palpation of the radial pulse will give a rough idea of blood pressure and heart rate. A palpable pulse at the radial artery implies a systolic pressure of at least 80 mmHg. Palpable pulses at the femoral and carotid arteries imply systolic pressures of at least 70 and 60 mmHg, respectively. Diagnosis of systemic hypotension will significantly affect the route of administration for drugs, particularly epinephrine. Drugs given subcutaneously in hypotensive individuals will probably be wholly ineffective. Pulse rate will also be important for distinguishing vasovagal response (bradycardia) from primary hypotension with reflex tachycardia.

Auscultation of the neck and lungs will help to differentiate laryngeal edema with stridorous inspiratory sounds in the neck from the bronchial expiratory wheezes of bronchospasm and the basilar rales, pops and crackles suggesting pulmonary edema.

Contrast reactions are unpredictable, unfamiliar and unnerving. Fortunately, they occur in a medical setting, and relatively straightforward diagnostic tools and therapies should facilitate excellent patient care.

> *Remember:*   Calm yourself.
>   Diagnose before you treat.
>   Be liberal with oxygen and IV fluids.

The uncomfortable but calm patient

Problems that may occur in the uncomfortable but calm patient include the following:

- urticaria – few or multiple hives;

- angioedema;

- diffuse erythema.

Urticaria

The most common reaction to contrast material is an anaphylactoid reaction limited to the skin and subcutaneous soft tissue. Local vasodilation causes erythema, and leaky capillaries are responsible for the raised wheal. Pruritus is the most prominent complaint, and scratching generally worsens symptoms. The lesions wax and wane and tend to occur in clusters.

> *History:*   acute onset of itching;
>   may have known allergies or previous episodes of
>   hives.
> *Physical examination:* red, raised weals which blanch with pressure;
>   patchy, symmetric involvement;
>   itching, often intense;
>   vital signs stable.

If urticaria are extensive, pay close attention to the patient's blood pressure and watch for signs and symptoms of hypotension, especially orthostatic hypotension.

Angioedema

Angioedema is akin to giant, deep hives. The edematous reaction involves deeper subcutaneous soft tissues and tends to affect regions of mucous membranes, including the throat and larynx. Gastrointestinal involvement can produce abdominal colic. Angioedema is usually asymmetric and not associated with pruritus.

> *History:*   sense of swelling or thickening about the face,
>   mouth, or throat;
>   itching usually absent.
> *Physical Examination:* ill-defined area of deep swelling;
>   mottled discoloration;
>   vital signs stable.

Pay close attention to the patient's airway, as angioedema commonly involves the mucous membranes of the pharynx and larynx. Laryngeal edema is angioedema of the larynx and hypopharynx.

Diffuse erythema

Erythema is caused by cutaneous vasodilation. Patients with diffuse erythema are at significant risk for severe hypotension due to systemic peripheral vasodilation. Increased capillary permeability and escape of fluid into the interstitial space may exacerbate low blood pressure. These patients are frequently minimally symptomatic initially, especially if lying down.

History:	may be minimally symptomatic initially; may complain of tightness around the mouth or eyes; may feel hot or flushed; itching is often absent.
Physical examination:	skin is mottled or diffusely red ('lobster red'); pulse and pressure are most often normal initially; breath sounds are normal; *check for orthostatic hypotension.*

The diffusely erythematous patient may appear to be completely stable acutely, yet there is a very real danger of delayed, severe hypotension. Maintain IV access and give IV fluids prophylactically while the patient is observed in the department. Be very wary of orthostatic hypotension as the patient is moved from the examination room to the observation area.

Orthostatic hypotension   This involves changes in pulse and pressure with changes in patient position from lying to sitting or from sitting to standing:

- an increase in heart rate of $\geq$ 10 beats/min;

- a fall in systolic blood pressure of $\geq$ 10 mmHg;

- a fall in diastolic blood pressure of $\geq$ 5 mmHg.

Orthostatic tachycardia   Patients with good vascular tone and reflexes may compensate for intravascular depletion by a considerable increase in heart rate to maintain blood pressure.

For the patient who is hypotensive in the supine or prone position, maneuvers to check for orthostatic changes are both unnecessary and dangerous.[6]

The anxious, agitated patient

Problems that may occur in the anxious, agitated patient include the following:

- airway or breathing problems:
    laryngeal edema;

bronchospasm;
pulmonary edema;

- anxiety reaction;

- hypoglycemia;

- rigors;

- hypertensive crisis;

- angina.

Airway or breathing problems

Laryngeal edema   Laryngeal edema is angioedema of the larynx and pharynx. The patient presents with a change in voice or with difficulty in breathing or swallowing.

History:	sudden or progressive onset of hoarseness or voice change;
	breathing or swallowing difficulties located in the neck;
	sense of a lump or swelling in the throat.
Physical examination:	anxious patient, usually sitting on the edge of the table;
	hoarse or soft voice, cough;
	inspiratory stridor – harsh, high-pitched squeaky sound centered in the neck.
	Note: voice may change to a whisper as airway compromise worsens.

Bronchospasm   Here the contraction of bronchial smooth muscle narrows large and small airway segments. It is identical to an asthma attack.

History:	sudden onset of chest tightness;
	shortness of breath;
	cough and wheezing;
	often patient has a history of similar attacks.
Physical examiation:	anxious patient, usually sitting on the edge of the table;
	wheezes initially more prominent on exhalation;
	as the process worsens, wheezes become audible in inspiration and exhalation.
	Note: wheezes may become quieter as spasm worsens.

Pulmonary edema   Paradoxically, this patient may not seem as ill initially because pulmonary edema progresses through several stages before the patient becomes highly symptomatic and physical signs appear.

Classically, pulmonary edema due to left-sided heart failure with venous backup presents with shortness of breath and tachypnea due to interstitial edema and decreased pulmonary compliance. In the setting of contrast administration and anaphylactoid reaction, vasodilation in the pulmonary bed may allow escape of plasma and red blood cells into the lung interstitium, and eventually into the alveoli, without concurrent cardiac failure. Finally, interstitial edema breaks through the alveolar lining and fluid, including red blood cells, pours into the alveoli. Auscultation then reveals moist rales and wheezes, and the patient may produce pink, frothy sputum.

History: variable, frequently slow, onset of chest tightness;
patient feels progressively more anxious.

Physical examination: initially may appear uncomfortable, sitting up;
will become more anxious and diaphoretic;
respiration is rapid:
    initial breath sounds may be normal;
    there are moist crackles and pops in the lung bases;
    wheezes may be heard as well;
blood-tinged, pink, frothy sputum;
pulse may be rapid – abnormal gallops or murmurs.

It is very difficult to determine whether the cause is cardiogenic or anaphylactoid, although the patient's age may provide some indication. This patient needs to be transferred to the emergency room or the intensive-care unit for more complete evaluation and treatment.

Anxiety reaction or panic attack

In an anxiety reaction, patient behavior and symptoms are not congruent with signs. They may be sitting up, agitated, or lying down clutching at their neck or chest. They may be completely unresponsive.

History: ill-defined complaints of closeness or chest tightness;
complaints of heart fluttering or pounding;
complaints of tingling around the mouth or the
    extremities;
may not talk or help with evaluation;
may appear unconscious.

Physical examination: normal;
pulse, blood pressure and respiration may be slightly
    to moderately elevated;
breath sounds are normal;
the physician, nurse or technologist may feel
    confused or frustrated by the incongruent findings;
patients may not seem to be motivated to help
    in their own care, and may answer questions
    tangentially or not at all.

Hypoglycemia

Patients not allowed oral intake (NPO), or with multiple examinations in one day, may describe a syndrome similar to panic attack.

History:	may feel faint, weak or dizzy;
	ill-defined sense of anxiety, paranoia or foreboding;
	usually diabetic, and the patient may recognize these symptoms.
Physical examination:	normal.

Rigors

This is a rare reaction to contrast material, not unlike the shakes or shivers associated with a febrile illness. The patient lies on the table exhibiting uncontrollable shaking. This is a self-limiting reaction that probably has a hypothalamic origin. A patient may be exhausted following such intense muscle activity and the reaction may be intense enough to initiate *angina*.

History:	sudden onset of uncontrollable shaking.
Physical examination:	severe shaking with chattering of teeth and even rattling of examination table;
	signs, including temperature, are normal.

Hypertensive crisis

This is an unusual reaction with sudden elevation of the blood pressure, usually over 120 mmHg diastolic. The patient may first complain of a pounding headache, or may be obtunded, confused or may have convulsions.

History:	sudden onset of severe headache, nausea, vomiting, focal neurologic deficits, or seizure;
	sudden change in mentation.
Physical examination:	bounding pulse;
	blood pressure > 120 mmHg diastolic;
	may have focal neurologic deficit including aphasia, paresis.

Hypertensive crisis in patients with pheochromocytoma   Patients suspected of harboring pheochromocytoma may rarely experience severe hypertension secondary to iodinated contrast administration or abdominal compression. In addition, patients with syndromes of familial multiple endocrine adenomatosis, neurofibromatosis or von Hippel-Lindau disease may have unsuspected pheochromocytomas.

Angina pectoris

This is characterized by poorly localized, squeezing chest discomfort. Its onset may be isolated or may be secondary to respiratory or vascular compromise.

History:	moderate discomfort;
	typically centered behind the sternum or in the jaw, arms, back or shoulders;
	unlikely to be first episode, and the patient may recognize the symptoms.

Physical examination: patient may be diaphoretic;
                                                      check pulse, heart sounds and blood pressure, which
                                                             will probably be normal.

The subdued or unresponsive patient

Problems that may occur in the subdued or unresponsive patient include the following:

- vasovagal reaction;

- hypotension with tachycardia;

- seizure.

Vasovagal reaction

This is classically a reaction of young to middle-aged men. Watch for excessive fear or anxiety and patients who are overly talkative or quiet prior to an examination. Anxiety or pain reflex causes decreased sympathetic activity and increased vagal tone, resulting in peripheral vasodilation and bradycardia. A heavy sigh or yawn may precede symptoms.

History: prodromal symptoms, such as warmth or nausea,
                     weakness, light-headedness, diaphoresis;
            fainting.

Physical examination: pallid, diaphoretic patient;
            cold cloth on forehead;
            classic low blood pressure with low heart rate
                  (less than 60 beats/min);
            consciousness may fluctuate.

This is typically a reaction of younger patients. If an older patient presents with low blood pressure and slow pulse, consider the possibility of anaphylactoid reaction complicated by beta-adrenergic-blocking medications.

Hypotension with tachycardia

Diffuse vasodilation causes lowering of systemic vascular resistance. Leaky capillary beds allow plasma to pour into the extravascular space, further lowering the blood pressure and causing reflex tachycardia.

History: patient becomes unresponsive or has fluctuating
                     consciousness;
            may be preceded by erythematous reaction.

Physical examination: diffuse erythema or pallor;
            pulse may be difficult to palpate;
            rapid heart rate (> 100 beats/min).

Seizures

Generalized convulsive seizures are not uncommon in the patient with a severe hypotensive reaction, and they are almost always self-limiting. In the patient with no previous history of seizure, further imaging work-up rarely uncovers a responsible lesion.

References

1. Cohan RH, Dunnick NR, Bashore TM. Treatment of reactions to radiographic contrast material. *American Journal of Roentgenology International* 1988; **151**: 263–70.

2. Bielory L, Kaliner MA. Anaphylactoid reactions to radiocontrast materials. *Anesthesiology Clinics* 1985; **23**: 97–118.

3. Katayama H, Yamaguchi K, Kozuka T *et al.* Adverse reactions to ionic and nonionic contrast media. *Radiology* 1990; **175**: 621–8.

4. Lasser EC. Contrast media for urography. In: Pollack H, ed. *Clinical urography.* Philadelphia, PA: W. B. Saunders & Co., 1990: 23–36.

5. Metcalfe DD. Anaphylaxis and urticaria in children and adults. In: Schocket AL, ed. *Clinical management of urticaria and anaphylaxis.* New York: Marcel Delekar, Inc., 1993: 1–20.

6. Willms JL, Schneiderman H, Algramati PS. *Physical diagnosis: bedside evaluation of diagnosis and function.* Baltimore, MD: Williams and Wilkins, 1994, p. 81.

Treatment of acute contrast reactions

William H. Bush Jr

Reactions to intravascular contrast media are generally classified as either systemic (idiosyncratic) or chemotoxic. Idiosyncratic (i.e. pseudoallergic, anaphylaxis-like, allergic-like and anaphylactoid) systemic reactions occur unpredictably and independently of the dose or concentration of the agent. Most of these anaphylactoid reactions are related to release of active mediators. Conversely, chemotoxic-type effects relate to dose, the molecular toxicity of each agent, and the physiochemical characteristics of the contrast agents (i.e. osmolality, viscosity, hydrophilicity, calcium-binding properties and sodium content). Some reactions to injection of contrast media (e.g. sudden cardiopulmonary arrest) are difficult to categorize specifically in either of the two major reaction types.[1-7]

Most acute reactions are minor and no treatment is required. Approximately 1–2 per cent of patients receiving conventional, higher-osmolality, ionic contrast media (HOCM) intravascularly will have a non-life-threatening, moderate reaction that requires some treatment for abatement. Moderate reactions to lower-osmolality, nonionic contrast media (LOCM) are reduced five-fold compared to those from HOCM.[8-12] Severe, life-threatening reactions can be expected in 0.06 to 0.4 per cent (pooled data 0.13) of patients receiving intravascular administration of HOCM.[13] Again, severe reactions occur much less frequently with LOCM, although they are not eliminated. Most serious life-threatening reactions occur in the immediate post-injection period. Delayed reactions (more than 30 min, but within 2 days of the injection) are surprisingly common (8–27 per cent), but are rarely serious and almost always mild in character.[9,14]

Reported *mortality rates* have varied from 1 in 13 000[15] to 1 in 169 000.[11] A commonly quoted mortality rate is 1 in 75,000.[16] The Katayama study[11] reported a low mortality rate (1:169 000) that was the same for both ionic and nonionic radiocontrast agents. In my opinion, the decrease in mortality reported over the past two decades reflects many factors, particularly education in specific treatment of the various reactions and the selective use of nonionic, lower-osmolality contrast media for those patients at higher risk of an adverse effect.[6,10,11,13,17-19] Not yet fully understood, and alarming to the radiologist, is the occurrence of severe, life-threatening anaphylactoid reactions to even small doses of intravascular nonionic LOCM.[20,21]

Severe systemic anaphylactoid reactions to *gadolinium agents* occur uncommonly. The rate of occurrence of serious reactions has varied in reports from 1 in 350 000 injections[22] to 1 in 10 000.[23] Asthma appears to be a risk factor.[22,24] Fatal reactions, although rare, have been reported following injection of gadopentetate dimeglumine.[25]

The precise *pathogenesis of systemic reactions* to contrast media is still incompletely understood.[4,5,7] Histamine, bradykinin and leukotrienes are well-accepted mediators of anaphylaxis, and vasoactive prostaglandins and the complement factors (C3a and C5a) are considered to be likely mediators (Lasser hypothesis).[26] Anaphylaxis is the term reserved for the immediate events that follow antigen-IgE-mediated release of mediators from mast cells and basophils. However, non-IgE-mediated reactions may result in the release of identical mediators with similar end-organ responses. Such reactions are often termed *anaphylactoid* because the clinical features and the induced biochemical alterations are indistinguishable from true anaphylaxis.[27] It appears that *non*-IgE mechanisms probably account for many, if not all, events involved in contrast-related idiosyncratic reactions.[28,29] Risk of an anaphylactoid reaction is increased in patients who have previously had a reaction to contrast media and those with asthma and allergies; it may also be increased in patients taking beta-blocking medication.[6,18]

Types of reactions

Acute reactions occurring after systemic administration of contrast media are quite variable, and include nausea or vomiting, scattered to extensive urticaria, laryngeal edema, bronchospasm, isolated hypotension with or without compensatory tachycardia (compensatory tachycardia may be lacking in patients taking beta-adrenergic blockers), hypotension and sinus bradycardia (vagal reaction), generalized systemic anaphylactoid reaction (which may include severe bronchospasm, laryngeal edema and hypotension), angina, hypertension, convulsions and cardiopulmonary arrest. These various reactions may occur either as an isolated manifestation or in a variety of combinations, and serious life-threatening reactions may occur without specific preliminary symptoms.[30] Acute airway obstruction and hypotension are the most threatening manifestations of anaphylactoid reactions.[28] A vagal reaction with hypotension and sinus bradycardia frequently occurs independently of contrast material administration.

Responding to a contrast reaction

Every radiologist administering contrast material must be prepared to deal with acute contrast reactions. Rooms in which contrast material injections are performed should have available the emergency drugs used in the initial treatment of a reaction, and emergency equipment should be either in the room or in an immediately accessible area. It is my recommendation that a list of drugs and their

Table 3.1   Acute reactions to contrast media: treatment outline

Urticaria:
  Mild urticaria and pruritus: observation
    H-1 antihistamine (e.g. diphenhydramine, 25–50 mg PO/IM/IV)
  Severe urticaria – *add*:
    IV fluids (normal saline, lactated Ringer's solution)
    Epinephrine (1:10 000): 1 mL (0.1 mg), IV slowly (e.g. over 2–5 min)
    H-2 antihistamine
      (e.g. cimetidine injectable, 300 mg, diluted to 20 mL, slowly IV) (pediatric 5–10
        mg/kg, diluted to 20 mL, slowly IV)
      or
      (e.g. ranitidine injectable, 50 mg, diluted to 20 mL, slowly IV) (pediatric use not
        established)

Bronchospasm (isolated):
  Oxygen by mask (6–10 L/min)
  Beta-2-agonist metered-dose inhaler (2–3 deep inhalations)
    (e.g. metaproterenol, terbutaline or albuterol)
    (or use nebulizer if available: albuterol 0.5% solution, 0.5 mL in 3 mL of normal
      saline, breathe through nebulizer tube for 8–10 min)
  Epinephrine:
    Normal blood pressure, stable bronchospasm:
      Subcutaneous: 1:1000, 0.1–0.2 mL (0.1–0.2 mg); may give 0.3 mg
      (pediatric: 0.01 mg/kg up to 0.3 mg maximum, (e.g. 0.1–0.2 mg subcutaneously)
    Progressive bronchospasm or decreased blood pressure:
      IV: 1:10 000, 1 mL (0.1 mg) slowly (e.g. over 2–5 min.) (pediatric: 0.01 mg/kg, IV)

Laryngeal edema:
  Oxygen by mask (6–10 L/min)
  Epinephrine
    IV: 1:10 000, 1mL (0.1 mg), slowly (e.g. over 2–5 min) (pediatric: 0.01 mg/kg)
    Subcutaneous if no IV access: 1:10 000, 0.1–0.2 mL (0.1–0.2 mg) (pediatric: 0.01
      mg/kg up to 0.3 mg maximum dose)

Hypotension (isolated):
  Elevate patient's legs
  Oxygen by mask (6–10 L/min)
  IV fluids (primary therapy): rapidly, normal saline or lactated Ringer's solution
  If unresponsive: vasopressor, e.g., epinephrine or dopamine, call Code
    Epinephrine: IV injection, 1:10 000 dilution, 1 mL (0.1 mg), slowly over 2–5 min
    IV solution, 1 mg in 250 mL 5% dextrose water solution, start at 4 µg/min
      (1 mL/min)

Vagal reaction (hypotension and bradycardia):
  Elevate patient's legs
  Oxygen by mask (6–10 L/min)
  IV fluids: rapidly, normal saline or lactated Ringer's solution
  Atropine: 0.6–1.0 mg IV, repeat after 3–5 min as needed up to 3 mg total (adults)
    (pediatric: 0.02 mg/kg IV; starting dose: minimum 0.1 mg, maximum 0.6 mg;
    may repeat to 2-mg total dose)

Table 3.1 *continued*

Anaphylactoid reaction (generalized systemic reaction):
  Suction, as needed
  Elevate patient's legs if hypotensive
  Oxygen (6–10 L/min)
  IV fluids: normal saline or Ringer's solution
  Epinephrine:
    (a generalized reaction usually has hypotension or incipient hypotension as a
      significant component, therefore, an *IV route* for administration is advised)
    IV: 1:10 000, 1 mL (0.1 mg) slowly (e.g. incrementally over 2–5 min) (pediatric:
      0.01 mg/kg, IV, to 0.1-mg dose)
    Note: Limit the amount of epinephrine in patients taking noncardioselective beta-adrenergic
      blocking drugs.
  Alternate drug therapy for severe reaction in patients taking beta-adrenergic
    blocking medication:
    Isoproterenol, 1:5000 solution for injection (0.2 mg/mL), IV, 1.0 mL diluted to 10
      mL with normal saline; 1 mL (20 μg) increments (*Note: this may cause hypotension*
      or arrhythmias)
    Glucagon, 1 to 5 mg IV bolus, followed by IV infusion of 5–15 μg/min (*Note: this*
      may cause hypotension)
  Antihistamines:
    H-1 blocker:
      (e.g. diphenhydramine 25–50 mg), IV (*Note this may exacerbate or cause hypotension*)
    H-2 blocker:
      (e.g. cimetidine injectable 300 mg, diluted to 20 mL, slowly IV) (pediatric: 5–10
        mg/kg, diluted, slowly)
      or
      (e.g. ranitidine injectable 50 mg, diluted to 20 mL, slowly IV) (pediatric use not
        established)
  Beta-2-agonist metered-dose inhaler (MDI) (for persistent bronchospasm) (2 or 3
    inhalations)
    (e.g. metaproterenol, terbutaline or albuterol)
    (or use nebulizer if available: 0.5% albuterol solution, 0.5 mL in 3 mL of normal
      saline, breathe through nebulizer tube for 8–10 min)
  Corticosteroids:
    hydrocortisone 200 mg IV; methylprednisolone 80 mg IV

Angina:
  Oxygen by mask (6–10 L/min)
  IV fluids: very slowly
  Nitroglycerin: 0.4 mg, sublingually, may repeat after 15 min
  Morphine: 2 mg, IV

Hypertension:
  Oxygen: (6–10 L/min)
  IV fluids: very slowly, primarily to maintain IV access
  Nitroglycerin:

Table 3.1 *continued*

---

orally, 0.4-mg tablet, sublingually
topically, 2% ointment: apply 1- to 2-inch strip to skin
If secondary to autonomic dysreflexia:
nifedipine, 10-mg capsule, punctured or chewed and the contents swallowed
(*Note:* nifedipine administered sublingually, because of its very poor sublingual
absorption and reported serious adverse effects, is no longer recommended as the
first-line drug for treatment of all hypertensive crises)
If secondary to pheochromocytoma: phentolamine 5 mg, IV slowly

Seizures:
Protect the patient
Airway: suction as needed; monitor the airway for obstruction by tongue
Oxygen by mask (6–10 L/min)
If caused by hypotension with or without bradycardia, treat per protocol
Uncontrolled: consider diazepam, 5 mg, IV

---

dosages for treating the various contrast reactions (such as those listed in Table 3.1) should be posted on the wall in each room where intravascular contrast medium is injected. One could either create a list, use the listings that accompany the American College of Radiology's *Manual on Contrast Media* (1998), or copy Table 3.1 from this chapter. The radiologist should be immediately available for at least the critical first 4–5 minutes following contrast injection, and should remain nearby for the next 30 to 45 minutes. All intravenous contrast injections should be made through a short needle-catheter assembly that should be left in place to ensure venous access in the event of a major reaction.

General principles of treating contrast reactions

The initial response should include six basic steps: check the patient's pulse; ensure an adequate airway; release any abdominal compression; elevate the patient's legs; start oxygen supplementation; and secure intravenous access. Talking with the patient as you check his or her pulse provides much initial information – breathing and mentation are assessed, an estimate of systolic blood pressure is obtained and pulse rate distinguishes reactive tachycardia from a vagal reaction (bradycardia). A palpable radial artery pulse approximates a minimum systolic pressure of 80–90 mmHg. If the patient appears hypotensive, elevation of his or her legs moves more intravascular fluid into the central circulatory system and enhances brain and heart perfusion.

Oxygen delivery by mask at a relatively high rate (6–10 L/min) is very important in the initial treatment of all moderate to severe reactions to intravascular contrast media and for those situations unrelated to contrast that occur in the radiology department (e.g. vagal reaction, hypotension, cardiac ischemia). Hypoxia is a major complicating factor that can adversely affect the function of drugs used for treatment of reactions, especially epinephrine. A 'partial nonrebreather' mask is optimal; nasal prongs are least effective in delivering good oxygenation. For acute contrast- or procedure-related reactions, oxygen should be used for all patients. A history of chronic obstructive pulmonary disease or emphysema is not a contraindication to the institution of oxygen therapy for an acute reaction.[31]

Intravascular fluid replacement is very important, and it has been reported to be the single most effective treatment for hypotension.[32] Early intervention with intravenous fluids, before starting drug therapy, should be re-emphasized as the highest priority in treating hypotension.[33] Normal saline or lactated Ringer's solution are preferred for acute, initial intravascular fluid expansion. Colloid solutions, such as 5 per cent human albumin, are selected if the hypotension is unresponsive to initial fluid therapy measures and the appropriate agents are available.[34]

For *drug therapy*, four main categories of drugs are utilized:

- antihistamines;

- steroids;

- adrenergic agonists;

- anticholinergics.

These are not listed in order of importance for treatment of a serious or severe reaction.[6]

Antihistamines (H-1-receptor antagonists) are the drugs most frequently used by radiologists to treat reactions to contrast media.[35] Although H-1 antihistamines are excellent for treating pruritus, they are of little value for treating the life-threatening manifestations of a severe contrast material reaction.[36,37] H-2-receptor antagonists (e.g. cimetidine) have been suggested for treatment of a severe reaction,[38] but this approach has not been supported by other investigators.[39] H-1- and H-2-receptor antagonists can be used as secondary drugs in the treatment of generalized systemic contrast reactions.[3,18,37] For the treatment of pruritus, an H-1-receptor blocker (e.g. diphenhydramine) is more effective than an H-2-receptor blocker (e.g. cimetidine) alone or combined as a dual therapy. For acute urticaria, the combination is more effective than an H-1-blocker alone.[40]

The use of *corticosteroids* for the initial treatment of acute, severe anaphylaxis is not supported by reliable experimental data. Large doses of intravenous corticosteroids are often given empirically to treat anaphylactoid reactions. However, their value is limited to longer-term stabilization and prevention of rebound of the anaphylactoid reaction because of their slow onset of action.[41–43]

Epinephrine has long been considered the drug of choice in treating acute anaphylactic reactions, yet no uniformly agreed upon regimen for its utilization in treating contrast reactions has been established.[3,39] The alpha-agonist effects of epinephrine increase blood pressure and reverse peripheral vasodilatation. These vasoconstrictive effects also decrease angioedema and urticaria.[44] The beta-agonist actions of epinephrine reverse bronchoconstriction, produce positive inotropic and chronotropic cardiac effects (an increase in the strength and rate of cardiac contractions), and may increase levels of intracellular cyclic adenosine monophosphate (AMP).[45,46] An increase in baseline cyclic AMP levels is generally considered to inhibit mediator release from inflammatory cells.[47,48]

Subcutaneous administration of 0.1–0.3 mg (0.1–0.3 mL) of 1:1000 aqueous epinephrine solution may be an effective treatment when there is an adequate peripheral circulation. However, if the circulation is poor or hypotension is developing, the subcutaneous route will probably be inadequate.[49] With subcutaneous injection, slowed absorption of epinephrine occurs because of its local vasoconstrictor effect, and a large subcutaneous dose of 0.5–1.5 mg (1:1000 concentration) may only give an absorbed dose of 10–30 μg/min.[46] Subcutaneous absorption is undependable and greatly influenced by the clinical condition of the patient. Absorption during maximal need may be insufficient and, conversely, large doses given subcutaneously or intramuscularly can be absorbed rapidly, particularly when hypotension is corrected, potentially causing an excess adrenergic effect.[50,51]

Intravenous epinephrine should be utilized whenever there is rapid progression of symptoms or when hypotension is suspected.[6,18,46,52–56] Initially, a low dose of 0.1 mg (1 mL) of 1:10,000 solution is given slowly over 2 to 5 mins. Following this initial low dose of IV epinephrine, additional small doses are given incrementally depending on the patient's response to the epinephrine. Epinephrine may also be administered as an aerosolized mist, endotracheally or transtracheally.[57,58] With endotracheal administration, the drug is usually absorbed rapidly in 5 to 10 breaths.[59] For endotracheal administration, most authorities recommend that the dose should be the same as that used intravenously.[49,59,60]

For infants and children, the subcutaneous dose of 1:1000 epinephrine is 0.01 mg/kg of body weight, up to a maximum of 0.3 mL (0.3 mg). For intravenous administration, a lower dose of 1:10 000 dilution is used (e.g. max. 0.1 mg).[34,37]

Epinephrine is an excellent, if not the best, drug for treating many serious contrast reactions. Its use necessitates careful attention and specific application. For example, in individuals with a fragile intracerebral or coronary circulation, the vasoconstrictive alpha-agonist effects of a *large dose* of epinephrine may invoke a hypertensive crisis or myocardial ischemia.[44] Beta-receptor sites ordinarily respond to lower doses of epinephrine than alpha-sites, but if a patient is on beta-blockers, the refractory response that may occur could encourage the radiologist to increase the dose of epinephrine to the point where unwanted alpha-effects would be generated. Patients with chronic asthma may simulate patients receiving beta-blockers, since a systemic beta-adrenergic hyporesponsiveness has long been documented in this group of patients.

Patients taking beta-blocking medications (e.g. propranolol) may require alternative drug therapy for a persisting, severe systemic anaphylactoid contrast reaction. *Isoproterenol*, because it is a pure beta-agonist, can override the beta block to achieve a beta-adrenergic effect without the problem of an unwanted excess alpha-adrenergic effect.[61] However, isoproterenol can cause arrhythmias or hypotension.[46,62] The dosage of isoproterenol is titrated to effect, diluting the 1:5000 solution to 10 mL and administering at 20 μg (1 mL)/min. Some epinephrine will probably be required to achieve the alpha-adrenergic effect of vasoconstriction and control of edema, although the epinephrine can be given at a low dose.[6] This combination of isoproterenol and smaller doses of epinephrine achieves the desired alpha- and beta-adrenergic effects while avoiding a high dose of epinephrine and excessive alpha-adrenergic effects. *Glucagon*, a catabolic peptide hormone that stimulates adenylate cyclase, is another option for the patient taking a beta-blocker who is having a persisting, severe anaphylactoid contrast reaction, because glucagon has both positive inotropic and chronotropic effects on the heart.[28] The dose of glucagon is 1–5 mg by IV bolus, followed by an intravenous infusion of 5–15 μg/min. Unlike isoproterenol, glucagon does not appear to cause arrhythmias but, like isoproterenol, it may cause hypotension.[63]

Epinephrine should be avoided, if possible, when treating a pregnant patient who is displaying a severe contrast reaction and hypotension.[64] Because the uterine vessels are sensitive to the alpha-adrenergic effects of epinephrine, the combination of hypotension plus epinephrine can cause serious sequelae to the fetus. Ephedrine (25–50 mg IV push) is suggested as an alternative medication.[64]

Atropine is the drug of choice for treating symptomatic bradycardia and for treating the vagal reaction (hypotension plus bradycardia) that is refractory to intravenous fluid therapy.[18,65–68] In the adult, a starting dose of 0.6–1.0 mg IV is strongly recommended, since lower doses may paradoxically worsen the bradycardia. Additional atropine may be given every 3–5 min for symptomatic bradycardia, up to a total dose of about 3.0 mg in adults, which approximates to the maximally vagolytic dose (0.04 mg/kg).[3,18,65–68] In adults, a transcutaneous pacemaker should be considered as one approaches the maximal dose of atropine if the bradycardia persists and the patient remains symptomatic.

The initial pediatric dose of atropine is 0.02 mg/kg up to a maximum 0.6-mg dose, with a Pediatric Advanced Life Support (PALS) recommended minimum starting dose of 0.1 mg. Recommended total dose in pediatrics is 1.0 mg for infants and 2.0 mg for adolescents.

Specific treatment plans

Table 3.1 and the following discussion summarize specific treatment plans for the more frequently observed adverse reactions.[6,18,52] However, these recommendations are not the only effective treatments.[19,69–71] Develop your own protocol, and review and update it periodically. Table 3.2 lists the drugs that I commonly use to treat acute contrast reactions. This selected group of medications is kept in a special kit (a tackle box stocked and maintained by the hospital pharmacy) in areas where contrast media is injected, so that these specific medications are readily available and easy to identify and select.

Table 3.2 Emergency contrast reaction treatment kit

Drug	Amount
Atropine 1 mg/mL vial	3
Beta-2-agonist metered-dose inhaler (e.g. metaproterenol 1.5% 10-mL inhaler) (single-use metered-dose inhaler)	1
Corticosteroid (e.g. methylprednisolone 80-mg vial)	1
Epinephrine (1:1000) 1 mg/mL vial	1
Epinephrine (1:10 000) 1 mg/10 mL (premixed, prepackaged emergency syringe)	1
H-1 antihistamine (e.g. diphenhydramine 50 mg/mL vial)	1
H-2 antihistamine (e.g. ranitidine 50 mg/2-mL vial)	1
Nifedipine 10-mg capsule	2
Nitroglycerin 2% ointment, tube; 0.4 mg tablet	1,2

Nausea and vomiting

Nausea and vomiting are usually self-limiting. However, they may also be early signs of more severe reactions. Lalli found that 20 per cent of fatal contrast reactions occurring in response to urographic examinations with HOCM began with nausea and vomiting.[72] For this reason, the patient should be observed closely for systemic symptoms, while maintaining intravenous access.

1 Position the patient to avoid aspiration.

2 Keep the patient under close observation (e.g. for 30 min).

Urticaria

For a few scattered hives or mild pruritus, treatment is usually not necessary. An H-1 antihistamine can be given to help to alleviate unpleasant symptoms of pruritus.[40] However, the patient should be observed closely for the development of other systemic symptoms, while maintaining intravenous access.

With diffuse erythema or extensive urticaria, leakage of fluid into the extravascular space with subsequent hypotension may occur. In such situations, treatment with IV fluids (e.g. normal saline) and small doses of IV epinephrine is recommended. IV epinephrine is very effective in reversing cutaneous reactions to intravascular contrast media.[37]

The following measures should be taken.

For *mild* urticaria:

1 observation until it is resolving;

For *moderate* urticaria:

1 administer H-1-receptor blocker (e.g. diphenhydramine, 25–50 mg, PO, IM or IV);

2 H-2-receptor blocker (e.g. cimetidine) may be added;[40]

3 observation until urticaria is resolving.

For *severe* urticaria, angioedema or diffuse erythema:

1 alpha-adrenergic agonist (low-dose epinephrine: 1.0 mL (0.1mg) 1:10 000, IV slowly over 2–5 mins; repeat as necessary);

2 IV fluids (normal saline or lactated Ringer's solution);

3 H-1-receptor blocker (e.g. diphenhydramine) plus H-2-receptor blocker (e.g. cimetidine);

4 corticosteroids IV (e.g. hydrocortisone 200 mg; prednisolone 100 mg; methyl-prednisolone 80 mg).[43,47,49]

Bronchospasm

Bronchospasm tends to occur in patients who already have a history of bronchospasm. The diagnosis depends on good auscultation of the lungs, which will reveal expiratory wheezes. Bronchospasm without coexisting cardiovascular problems should be treated with oxygen and inhaled bronchodilators. Inhaled beta-2-adrenergic agonists such as albuterol, metaproterenol and terbutaline deliver large doses of bronchodilating beta-2-agonist drugs directly to the airways, with minimal systemic absorption and therefore minimal cardiovascular effect. A nebulizer, although not often available in most radiology departments, is an excellent method for delivery of bronchodilating agents. Disposable metered-dose inhalers (MDI) containing a beta-2-agonist drug are readily available and easily stocked as a routine medication in areas where contrast is injected. Treatment with an MDI typically involves two or three deep inhalations. Aminophylline is no longer a 'first-line' drug, having been supplanted by the beta-agonist inhalers. Furthermore, aminophylline may cause significant hypotension. If the initial beta-agonist inhaler treatment is not fully effective, add nebulized beta-agonist medication (e.g. nebulized albuterol solution) or administer IV epinephrine. Epinephrine is indicated for treating bronchospasm that is unrelieved by inhaled bronchodilators.

Treatment options can be summarized as follows:

1 oxygen delivered by mask (6–10 L/min);

2 beta-2 agonist inhaler (e.g. albuterol) (metered-dose inhaler or nebulized);

3 IV epinephrine (1:10 000).

Laryngeal edema

Patients with laryngeal edema may present with hoarseness or coughing. Severe cases will result in inspiratory stridor (a preponderance of 'sounds' heard at the neck) and severe or increasing respiratory distress. Quick and correct treatment is essential. Laryngeal edema does not respond well to inhaled beta-agonists, and in fact these agents may actually worsen the edema. Laryngeal edema should be treated with IV epinephrine. Therefore, clinical evaluation and auscultation of the patient prior to beginning treatment are extremely important for differentiating laryngeal edema from bronchospasm.

Epinephrine is the primary treatment for laryngeal edema. If hypotension is present or developing, subcutaneously administered medication may not be absorbed adequately to achieve an optimum systemic effect. Intravenous epinephrine should be utilized whenever symptoms are progressing rapidly or hypotension is suspected or imminent.[6,18,46,53,54]

Treatment options can be summarized as follows:

1 oxygen delivered by mask (6–10 L/min);

2 IV epinephrine (1:10 000), 1.0 mL (0.1 mg) administered slowly over 2–5 mins, and repeated as needed. For children, begin with a subcutaneous dose of 1:1000 epinephrine (0.01 mg/kg) (0.01 mL/kg up to 0.03 mL maximum) because veins are often difficult to find.

Isolated hypotension

Profound hypotension may occur without respiratory symptoms. Tachycardia, or possibly a normal cardiac rate, helps to differentiate this reaction from the vagal reaction (hypotension plus sinus bradycardia). In patients who have been taking beta-adrenergic-blocking medications (e.g. propranolol), compensatory tachycardia may not occur in response to hypotension. Isolated hypotension is best treated initially by rapid intravenous fluid replacement (e.g. normal saline, lactated Ringer's solution), reserving vasopressor drugs for those patients who are refractory to fluid therapy.[33,34] Elevation of the patient's legs is very important. This simple maneuver returns about 700 mL of blood to the central circulation immediately, and is preferable to placing the patient in the Trendelenburg position.[45] Remove any abdominal compression (e.g. that applied during excretory urography). Supplementary oxygen should be administered. If the response to aggressive IV fluid therapy is ineffective, then addition of a catecholamine vasoconstrictor should be considered (i.e. IV epinephrine or IV dopamine).

Treatment can be summarized as follows:

1 elevate the patient's legs;

2 oxygen delivery by mask (6–10 L/min);

3 IV fluids (normal saline, lactated Ringer's solution);

4 secondary measures: vasopressor drug, e.g. epinephrine. Epinephrine, 1:10 000, 1 mL (0.1 mg) given slowly over 2–5 min; IV drip infusion, 1–4 μg/min;[31,49] the rate can be increased to 5–20 μg/min.[57]

5 if response to initial therapy is poor, call a Code.

Vagal reaction

This adverse response to the injection of a contrast medium, or to painful or anxiety-provoking procedures, is characterized by sinus bradycardia and hypotension. Its exact cause is unknown. The reaction initially causes vasodilatation with expansion of the intravascular space, and excess vagal activity causes bradycardia. Elevation of the patient's legs and rapid infusion of intravenous fluids will successfully reverse the reaction in most patients. Intravenous atropine, to block vagal stimulation of the cardiac conduction system, should be administered to those patients whose hypotension is refractory to fluid therapy. Because small doses of atropine can be detrimental and exacerbate the bradycardia associated with a contrast medium-induced vagal reaction,[65,66,68] larger doses (0.6–1.0 mg) are indicated. My recommendation is that 1.0 mg be given IV (slow push) as the initial dose, and additional doses of 0.6–1.0 mg be given every 3 to 5 minutes as needed to correct the bradycardia, up to a total dose of 3 mg in adults.[3,6] For pediatric patients, the initial IV dose is 0.02 mg/kg, with a minimum starting dose of 0.1 mg and a maximum starting dose of 0.6 mg; this may be repeated up to a total dose of 2 mg.

If the bradycardia is refractory to vagolytic doses of atropine, transcutaneous cardiac pacing may be required.

Treatment can be summarized as follows:

1 elevate the patient's legs;

2 IV fluids (e.g. normal saline, lactated Ringer's solution);

3 oxygen delivered by mask;

4 IV atropine; in adults, 0.6–1.0 mg, repeated as necessary up to a total dose of 3 mg to correct persistent symptomatic bradycardia.

Systemic anaphylactoid reactions

These are acute, rapidly progressing generalized systemic reactions characterized by multisystem involvement with pruritus, urticaria, angioedema, respiratory distress (bronchospasm, laryngeal edema) and profound hypotension. These reactions require prompt treatment. Initial treatment includes maintenance of an airway, administration of oxygen, rapid infusion of intravenous fluids, and administration of adrenergic medications.

Epinephrine is the drug of choice and should be administered intravenously for prompt, effective action and to avoid suboptimal absorption from subcutaneous tissues due to developing hypotension.[3,6,18,44–46,53–56] A low dose, 1.0 mL (0.1 mg) of 1:10 000 solution, is given at a relatively slow rate (over 2 to 5 min) and is titrated to effect.[6,44,45,56] If the reaction does not respond to this initial, slowly administered, low IV dose, increase the rate of injection.[34,37,57]

Intravenous epinephrine should be given with caution to elderly patients or hypoxic patients, in whom there is increased risk of severe cardiac arrhythmias. In addition, the amount of intravenous epinephrine should be limited in patients who are receiving noncardioselective beta-blocking medications (e.g. propranolol) (see discussion above).

When the use of epinephrine is inadvisable, bronchospasm can be treated with a beta-2-agonist inhaler and hypotension can be treated with intravenous fluids. For a patient on beta-blockers who is having a severe generalized anaphylactoid reaction that has not responded to beta-2 agonist inhalers, IV fluids and the initial small dose of IV epinephrine, *isoproterenol* can be considered. Isoproterenol is a pure beta-agonist (both beta-1 and beta-2) with no alpha effects and can be used to 'override' the beta blockade. The appropriate dosage can be titrated to effect, diluting the 1:5000 solution to 10 mL and administering it at 20 μg (1 mL)/min. Isoproterenol is also a potent drug, and can cause hypotension and arrhythmias.[46,62] A small amount of IV 1:10 000 epinephrine should be given to the patient to achieve some alpha effect (vasoconstriction) and to correct laryngeal edema and angioedema.[6] Another option for treatment of a severe reaction in the patient taking beta-blockers is *glucagon*, because of its positive inotropic and chronotropic effects on the heart.[61] The cardiac stimulant effects of glucagon are not associated with increased myocardial irritability, in contradistinction to isoproterenol.[63] The dose of glucagon is 1–5 mg by IV bolus, followed by an intravenous infusion of 5–15 μg/min.[28] Like isoproterenol, glucagon may cause hypotension.

Treatment can be summarized as follows:

1 call for assistance;

2 administer oxygen by mask (6–10 L/min);

3 IV fluids (e.g. normal saline, lactated Ringer's solution);

4 IV epinephrine (1:10 000), 1 mL (0.1 mg), administered slowly over 2–5 min and repeated as needed;

5 secondary measures – antihistamines, corticosteroids;

6 options for patients taking beta-blockers – glucagon, isoproterenol.

Pulmonary edema/angina

Patients with pulmonary edema are usually very anxious and very short of breath due to reduced pulmonary compliance. The cardinal auscultatory signs are crackles or rales at the lung bases. Cardiac monitoring is important. Patients with pulmonary edema may not respond rapidly to treatment, and transfer to an emergency room or intensive-care unit early in treatment is recommended.

1 Sit the patient up if possible; elevate the patient's head.

2 Administer oxygen by mask (6–10 L/min).

3 Perform electrocardiographic monitoring.

4 Consider nitroglycerin, furosemide (Lasix®) and morphine.

Hypertensive crisis

This is encountered more commonly as an autonomic dysreflexic response during an examination such as cystography in a spinal injury patient (spinal injury above T-6) or during renal angioplasty. The patient may complain of a 'pounding' headache or angina, or may have few complaints. Controversy exists about which drug is most appropriate for treating an acute hypertensive reaction.[73,74] For the hypertensive episode caused by autonomic dysreflexia, some authors consider nifedipine to be the drug of choice; the 10-mg capsule is punctured or bitten and the contents are swallowed.[74] The dose may be repeated after 30 min. For others, nitroglycerin is recommended as the drug of choice for treating a hypertensive reaction or crises, and nifedipine is no longer advocated.[73] Absorption of nifedipine occurs not via the sublingual route but through the gastrointestinal tract, and the blood-pressure response to biting a capsule or dripping the contents sublingually may be delayed or unpredictable.[73] Nitroglycerin is given sublingually as a 0.4-mg tablet, which usually has a duration of 10–30 minutes, or as a topically applied 2 per cent ointment. A 1- to 2-inch strip of ointment is applied and rubbed into the skin, and its duration of effect is 3–6 h.[73] Nitroglycerin can also be given IV as a bolus dose of 100–200 μg, with maintenance infusion titrated to effect; duration effect is very brief (< 5 min). If pheochromotoma is suspected as a cause of the hypertension, phentolamine IV is the drug of choice.

Treatment can be summarized as follows:

1 administer oxygen by mask (6–10L/min);

2 nitroglycerin: either as a nitroglycerin tablet sublingually, topical application of a 1- to 2-inch strip of 2 per cent ointment or IV at 100–200 μg;

3 call for assistance;

4 for hypertension related to autonomic dysreflexia, administer nifedipine (e.g. Procardia®) as a 10-mg capsule, ask patient to puncture or bite capsule and swallow its contents (alternatively, consider nitroglycerin 0.4 mg sublingual);

5 for hypertension caused by pheochromocytoma, administer phentolamine (e.g. Regitine®), 5 mg, IV.

Seizures/convulsions

Seizures are often due to a severe hypotensive reaction (e.g. profound vagal reaction). For these patients, therapy is directed at protecting the patient (e.g. turn them on their side to prevent aspiration). Evaluate the patient for hypotension as a cause, so that treatment is specific and appropriate with IV fluids, oxygen and IV atropine if bradycardia is present. Seizures may also be due to the contrast medium irritating an underlying abnormal focus in the brain, or may be incidental.

Treament can be summarized as follows:

1 avoid aspiration by the patient;

2 administer oxygen by mask (6–10 L/min);

3 treat hypotension or vagal reaction if present;

4 administer IV diazepam (e.g. Valium®), 5 mg, if the seizure is caused by known irritative focus, or if seizure activity is prolonged; titrate to cessation of seizure and monitor respiration carefully.[59,75]

Diabetic hypoglycemia

This is not in fact a reaction to the contrast medium, but is often a result of the preparation (e.g. no oral intake) for an examination or procedure. The patient may complain of vague symptoms such as not feeling well, lightheadedness, or blurred thinking. If in doubt, and a hypoglycemic state is possible, prompt administration of IV dextrose (50 per cent dextrose, 25 gm) is harmless and can help to stabilize these diabetic patients.

Treatment can be summarized as follows:

1 administer oxygen by mask;

2 IV fluids, D_5W;

3 give the patient a glass of juice or milk;

4 dextrose, 50 per cent solution, IV bolus.

Anxiety reaction

An anxiety reaction is a diagnosis of exclusion. If no abnormality is found after examining the patient's skin, listening to the lungs and evaluating the vital signs, one should consider panic attack as the possible cause of sense of shortness of breath, lightheadedness or anxiety. Certainly a cardiac cause of the symptoms is the diagnosis that needs to be excluded.

1 Monitor and reassure the patient.

2 Calm the patient.

3 Give the patient a paper bag to breathe into if there is hyperventilation (do not use if patient is hypoxic).

Cardiovascular collapse/cardiac arrest

Cardiac arrest is defined as occurring when the patient is unconscious, unresponsive and has no detectable pulse or blood pressure. If a patient is found in this condition, a 'Code' should be called and immediate cardiopulmonary resuscitation (CPR) should be started.[31,76]

Treatment can be summarized as follows:

1 call a Code;

2 start basic life support and CPR;

3 start cardiac monitoring as soon as equipment is available;

4 start defibrillation if appropriate; defibrillation supersedes CPR when the necessary equipment is available.

Summary

Prompt recognition of the type of reaction and initiation of specific treatment are vital. Evaluate the patient in an efficient, systematic manner. The earlier a reaction is recognized, identified, and treated, the better the outcome. Simple basic steps such as ensuring good oxygenation, evaluating the patient's pulse, elevating the patient's legs, and administering IV fluids may alone correct some reactions. Never rush to take immediate action using drugs until you have a clear understanding of the exact nature of the reaction. Conversely, do not delay or withhold the early administration of a critical medication such as IV epinephrine. Adequate preparation is the key.

References

1. Swanson DP, Shetty PC, Kastan DJ, Rollins N. Angiographic contrast media. In: Swanson D, Chilton H, Thrall J, eds. *Pharmaceuticals in medical imaging.* New York: Macmillan, 1990, 13–39.

2. Thrall JH. Adverse reactions to contrast media: etiology, incidence, treatment, prevention. In: Swanson DP, Chilton HM, Thrall JH eds., *Pharmaceuticals in medical imaging.* New York: Macmillan, 1990: 253–77.

3. Bush WH, Swanson DP. Acute reactions to intravascular contrast media: types, risk factors, recognition, and specific treatment. *American Journal of Roentgenology* 1991; **157**: 1153–61.

4. Lieberman P. Anaphylactoid reactions to radiocontrast material. *Immunology and Allergy Clinics* 1992; **12**: 649–70.

5. Almen T. The etiology of contrast medium reactions. *Investigative Radiology* 1994; **29** (Supplement 1), S37–S45.

6. Bush WH. Risk factors, prophylaxis and therapy of X-ray contrast media reactions. *Advances in X-ray Contrast* 1996; **3**: 44–53.

7. Spinazzi A, Davies A, Rosati G. Predictable and unpredictable adverse reactions to uroangiographic contrast media. *Academic Radiology* 1996; **3**: 5210–13.

8. Davies P, Roberts MB, Roylance J. Acute reactions to urographic contrast media. *British Medical Journal* 1975; **2**: 434–7.

9. McCullough M, Davies P, Richardson R. A large trial of intravenous Conray 325 and Niopam 300 to assess immediate and delayed reactions. *British Journal of Radiology* 1989; **62**: 260–65.

10. Wolf GL, Arenson RL, Cross AP. A prospective trial of ionic vs. nonionic contrast agents in routine clinical practice: comparison of adverse effects. *American Journal of Roentgenology* 1989; **152**: 939–44.

11. Katayama H, Yamaguchi K, Kozuka T, Takashima T, Seez P, Matsuura K. Adverse reactions to ionic and nonionic contrast media: a report from the Japanese Committee on the Safety of Contrast Media. *Radiology* 1990; **175**: 621–8.

12. Caro JJ, Trindade E, McGregor M. The risks of death and of severe nonfatal reactions with high- vs. low-osmolality contrast media: a meta-analysis. *American Journal of Roentgenology* 1991; **156**: 825–32.

13. Lawrence V, Matthai W, Hartmaier S. Comparative safety of high-osmolality and low-osmolality radiographic contrast agents. Report of a multidisciplinary working group. *Investigative Radiology* 1992; **27**: 2–28.

14. Yoshikawa H. Late adverse reactions to non-ionic contrast media. *Radiology* 1992; **183**: 737–40.

15. Shehadi WH. Death following intravascular administration of contrast media. *Acta Radiologica: Diagnosis* 1985; **26**: 457–61.

16. Hartman GW, Hattery RR, Witten DM, Williamson B. Mortality during excretory urography: Mayo Clinic experience. *American Journal of Roentgenology* 1982; **139**: 919–22.

17. Siegle RL. Rates of idiosyncratic reactions. Ionic versus nonionic contrast media. *Investigative Radiology* 1993; **28** (Supplement 5): S95–S98.

18. Bush WH, McClennan BL, Swanson DP. Contrast media reactions: prediction, prevention and treatment. *Postgraduate Radiology* 1993; **13**: 137–47.

19. McClennan BL. Adverse reactions to iodinated contrast media. Recognition and response. *Investigative Radiology* 1994; **29** (Supplement 1) : S46–S50.

20. Curry N, Schabel S, Reiheld C *et al*. Fatal reactions to intravenous nonionic contrast material. *Radiology* 1991; **178** : 361–2.

21. Baltaoglu G, Balkanci R, Tirnaksiz B. Fatal reaction after intra-arterial injection of nonionic contrast medium (letter). *American Journal of Roentgenology* 1994; **162**: 231.

22. Shellock R, Hahn H, Mink J *et al*. Adverse reaction to intravenous gadoteridol. *Radiology* 1993; **189**: 151–2.

23. Murphy K, Brunberg J, Cohan R. Adverse reaction to gadolinium contrast media: a review of 36 cases. *American Journal of Roentgenology* 1996; **167**: 847–9.

24. Nelson K, Gifford L, Lauber-Huber C *et al*. Clinical safety of gadopentetate dimeglumine. *Radiology* 1995; **196**: 439–42.

25. Jordan R, Mintz R. Fatal reaction to gadopentetate dimeglumine. *American Journal of Roentgenology* 1995; **164**: 743–4.

26. Lasser EC. Contrast media for urography. In: Pollack HM, ed. *Clinical urography*. Philadelphia, PA: W.B. Saunders & Co., 1990: 23–36.

27. Sheffer A. Anaphylaxis. *Journal of Allergy and Clinical Immunology* 1985; **75**: 227–33.

28. Winbery SL, Lieberman PL. Anaphylaxis. *Immunology and Allergy Clinics of North America* 1995; **15**: 447–76.

29. Genovese A, Stellato C, Marsella C *et al*. Role of mast cells, basophils and their mediations in adverse reactions to general anesthetics and radiocontrast media *International Archives of Allergy and Immunology* 1996; **110**: 13–22.

30. Bush WH, Swanson DP. Radiocontrast. *Immunology and Allergy Clinics of North America* 1995; **15**: 597–612.

31. Grauer K, Cavallaro D. *ACLS: certification preparation and a comprehensive review. (Volumes. I and II)*. St. Louis, MO: Mosby, Lifeline, 1993.

32. Obeid A, Johnson L, Potts J, et al. Fluid therapy in severe systemic reaction to radiopaque dye. *Annals of Internal Medicine* 1975; **83**: 317–21.

33. van Sonnenberg E, Neff CC, Pfister RC. Life-threatening hypotensive reactions to contrast media administration: comparison of pharmacologic and fluid therapy. *Radiology* 1987; **162**: 15–19.

34. Perkin RM, Anas NG. Mechanisms and management of anaphylactic shock not responding to traditional therapy. *Annals of Allergy* 1985; **54**: 201–8.

35. Lasser EC, CC Berry, LB Talner *et al*. Pretreatment with corticosteroids to alleviate reactions to intravascular contrast media. *New England Journal of Medicine* 1987; **317**: 845–9.

36. Goldberg M. Systemic reactions to intravascular contrast media – a guide for the anesthesiologist. *Anesthesiology* 1984; **60**: 46–56.

37. Yunginger JW. Anaphylaxis. *Current Problems in Pediatrics* 1992; **22**: 130–46.

38. Mayumi H, Kimura S, Asano M. Intravenous cimetidine as an effective treatment for systemic anaphylaxis and acute allergic skin reactions. *Annals of Allergy* 1987; **50**: 447–51.

39. Kelly JS, Prielipp RC. Is cimetidine indicated in the treatment of acute anaphylactic shock? (letter). *Anesthesia and Analgesia* 1990; **71**: 100–106.

40. Runge JW, Martinez JC, Caravati EM, Williamson SG, Hartsell SC. Histamine antagonists in the treatment of acute allergic reactions. *Annals of Emergency Medicine* 1992; **21**: 237–42.

41. Lasser EC, Lang J, Sovak M, Kolb W, Lyon S, Hamlin AE. Steroids: theoretical and experimental basis for utilization in prevention of contrast media reactions. *Radiology* 1977; **125**: 1–9.

42. Greenberger PA, Halwig TM, Patterson R *et al.* Emergency administration of a radiocontrast media in high-risk patients. *Journal of Allergy and Clinical Immunology* 1986; **77**: 630–35.

43. Netzel MC. Anaphylaxis: clinical presentation, immunologic mechanisms, and treatment. *Journal of Emergency Medicine* 1986; **4**: 227–36.

44. Barach EM, Nowak RM, Tennyson GL, Tomlanovich MC. Epinephrine for treatment of anaphylactic shock. *Journal of the American Medical Association* 1984; **251**: 2118–22.

45. Smith NT, Corbascio A. The use and misuse of pressor agents. *Anesthesiology* 1970; **33**: 58–101.

46. Hoffman BB, Lefkowitz RJ. Catecholamines and sympathomimetic drugs. In: Gilman AG, Rall TW, Nies AS, Taylor P, eds. *The pharmacological basis of therapeutics*. New York: McGraw-Hill Publishers, 1990: 192–8.

47. Ignarro L, Colombo C. Enzyme release from polymorphonuclear leukocyte lysosomes: regulation by autonomic drugs and cyclic nucleotides. *Science* 1973; **180**: 1181–3.

48. Zurier R, Weissmann G, Hoffstein S *et al.* Mechanisms of lysosomal enzyme release from human leukocytes. II. Effects of cAMP and cGMP, autonomic agonists, and agents which affect microtubule function. *Journal of Clinical Investigation* 1974; **53**: 297–309.

49. Stoloff R, Adams SL, Orfan N, Harris KE, Greenberger PA, Patterson R. Emergency medical recognition and management of idiopathic anaphylaxis. *Journal of Emergency Medicine* 1992; **10**: 693–8.

50. Ferry DR, Henry RL, Kern MJ. Epinephrine-induced myocardial infarction in a patient with angiographically normal coronary arteries. *American Heart Journal* 1986; **111**: 1193–5.

51. Saff R, Nahhas A, Fink JN. Myocardial infarction induced by coronary vasospasm after self-administration of epinephrine. *Annals of Allergy* 1993; **70**: 396–8.

52. Harris JB, Bush WH. How to treat adverse reactions to contrast media. *Contemporary Urology* 1996; **8**: 33–46.

53. Bush WH, McClennan BL. Treatment of adverse contrast media reaction (letter). *Radiology* 1995; **194**: 289.

54. Bush WH, McClennan BL. Epinephrine administration for severe adverse reactions to contrast agents (letter). *Radiology* 1995; **196**: 879.

55. Sadler DJ, Parrish F, Coulthard A. Contrast media reactions (letter). *Clinical Radiology* 1995; **50**: 506.

56. Barach EM. Epinephrine for anaphylactic shock (letter). *Journal of the American Medical Association* 1985; **253**: 510–11.

57. Mueller U, Mosbech H, Blaauw P et al. Emergency treatment of allergic reactions to hymenoptera stings. *Clinical and Experimental Allergy* 1991; **21**: 281–8.

58. Ewan PW. Route of administration of adrenaline for the treatment of anaphylactic reaction to bee or wasp stings (letter). *Clinical and Experimental Allergy* 1992; **22**: 753–6.

59. Powers RD, Donowitz LG. Endotracheal administration of emergency medications. *Southern Medical Journal* 1984; **77**: 340–41.

60. Roberts JR, Greenberg ME Baskin SI. Endotracheal epinephrine in cardiorespiratory collapse. *Journal of the American College of Emergency Physicians* 1979; **8**: 515.

61. Ingall M, Goldman G, Page LB. Beta-blockade in stinging insect anaphylaxis (letter). *Journal of the American Medical Association* 1984; **251**: 432.

62. Steen PA, Tinkler JH, Pluth JR et al. Efficacy of dopamine, dobutamine and epinephrine during emergence from cardiopulmonary bypass in man. *Circulation* 1978; **57**: 378–85.

63. Lvoff R, Wilcken DEL. Glucagon in heart failure and in cardiogenic shock. *Circulation* 1972; **45**: 534–9.

64. Entman SS, Moise KJ. Anaphylaxis in pregnancy. *Southern Medical Journal* 1984; **77**: 402.

65. Stanley RJ, Pfister RC. Bradycardia and hypotension following use of intravenous contrast media. *Radiology* 1976; **121**: 5–7.

66. Chamberlain DA, Turner P, Sneddon JM. Effects of atropine on heart rate in healthy man. *Lancet* 1967; **2**: 12–15.

67. Fischer HW, Colgan FJ. Causes of contrast media reactions. *Radiology* 1976; **121**: 223.

68. Brown JH. Atropine, scopolamine, and antimuscarinic drugs. In: Gilman AG, Rall TW, Nies AS, Taylor P, eds. *The pharmacological basis of therapeutics*. New York: McGraw-Hill Publishers, 1990: 150–65.

69. Siegle RL, Lieberman P. A review of untoward reactions to iodinated contrast material. *Journal of Urology* 1978; **119**: 581–7.

70. Cohan RH, Dunnick NR. Treatment of reactions to radiologic contrast material. *American Journal of Roentgenology* 1988; **151**: 263–7.

71. Cohan RH, Leder RA, Ellis JH. Treatment of adverse reactions to radiographic contrast media in adults. *Radiologic Clinics of North America* 1996; **34**: 1055–60.

72. Lalli AF. Contrast media reactions: data analysis and hypothesis. *Radiology* 1980; **134**: 1–12.

73. Grossman E, Messerli FH, Grodzicki T, Kowey P. Should a moratorium be placed on sublingual nifedipine capsules given for hypertensive emergencies and pseudoemergencies? *Journal of the American Medical Association* 1996; **276**: 1328–31.

74. Braddom RL, Rocco JF. Autonomic dysreflexia. A survey of current treatment. *American Journal of Physical Medicine and Rehabilitation* 1991; **70**: 234–41.

75. Delgado-Escueta AV, Wasterlain C, Treiman DM *et al*. Management of status epilepticus. *New England Journal of Medicine* 1982; **306**: 1337–40.

76. Emergency Cardiac Care Committee and Subcommittees, American Heart Association. Guidelines for cardiopulmonary resuscitation and emergency cardiac care. III. Adult advanced cardiac life support. *Journal of the American Medical Association* 1992; **268**: 2199–241.

4 Pediatric contrast reactions and airway management

Jane S. Matsumoto and John T. Wald

Contrast media in children

Children show fewer reactions to intravenous contrast material than adults, and they tend to have anaphylactoid reactions rather than primary cardiac problems. In general, children have healthy hearts, in contrast to the elderly patients who are often seen in radiology departments. In the pediatric population, cutaneous and respiratory reactions predominate.

The usual recommended dose for intravenous iodinated contrast media is 1 mL/lb, or 2.2 mL/kg, up to a maximum dose of 100 mL. For high-osmolality contrast media (HOCM), the minor anaphylactoid reaction rate is 3 per cent and for lower-osmolality contrast media (LOCM), the rate drops to 0.9 per cent.[1-4] In addition to a lower rate of anaphylactoid reactions, LOCM has the added benefit of causing less nausea and vomiting and decreasing the morbidity from soft tissue extravasation.[5] Both are important factors in small children who may be restrained, sedated, or have small veins with tenuous IV access. LOCM is recommended for children who are less than 1 year old, sedated, restrained, have a history of allergies or asthma, have cardiac or renal disease, or are critically ill. Many radiology departments use LOCM for all children. Because of the potential risk of contrast reactions, intravenous access should be maintained in radiology patients until the examination has been completed.

The most common adverse reactions to intravenous contrast material in children are nausea and vomiting. Therefore, it is important to have the child fasting with an empty stomach. This is especially true in the case of the sedated or restrained child. The optimal fasting state requires withholding of solids for 4 to 6 h and withholding of clear liquids for 2 h before the examination. Cow's milk and formula are considered to be solids, and breast milk is considered to be a clear liquid.

Contrast reactions and treatment

Hives are a common anaphylactoid reaction, and may develop immediately or over the course of 1 h after contrast injection. Other minor reactions include bullae, rhinorrhea and sneezing. Alert observation is very important in caring for infants and young children, because they often cannot or will not verbalize discomfort or problems. Cutaneous reactions may be best appreciated if the child is wearing a gown, so that any skin changes are more easily detected. The radiology staff must be alert to subtle physical changes in children.

Treatment for minor reactions is usually symptomatic, utilizing H-1 antihistamines such as diphenhydramine (Benadryl®) 1–2 mg/kg, IV or PO, up to a maximum dose of 50 mg. If the reaction is extensive or increasing, epinephrine may be needed. Epinephrine (1:1000) may be administered subcutaneously at a dose of 0.01 mL/kg up to 0.3 mL. The patient should be observed until symptoms and signs have resolved.

Significant respiratory reactions, such as bronchospasm and laryngeal edema, occur less commonly. Mild or moderate bronchospasm should be treated with a beta-2-agonist inhaler, such as an albuterol metered-dose inhaler. Two puffs may be given directly or through a 'spacer.' This can be repeated every 15–30 min as needed. For refractory bronchospasm or laryngeal edema, high-flow oxygen should be delivered, IV access needs to be secured, and backup emergency help should be summoned. Intravenous epinephrine (1:10 000) at a dose of 0.1 mL/kg (0.01 mg/kg) should be administered slowly and titrated to effect. This can be repeated as necessary every 5 min. If IV access has been lost, subcutaneous epinephrine (1:1000) at a dose of 0.01 mL/kg can be given as an alternative until IV access is re-established. IV steroids such as methylprednisolone (Solu-medrol®) at a loading dose of 2 mg/kg, although not effective immediately, can be given in order to provide longer term stabilization.

Anaphylaxis-like shock may occur in isolation or in combination with cutaneous or respiratory reactions. Emergency help should be summoned immediately. Initial treatment includes high-flow oxygen by mask and delivery of isotonic intravenous fluids, either normal saline or lactated Ringer's solution, in volumes of 20–40 mL/kg. Intravenous epinephrine (1:10 000 dilution) should be given at a dose of 0.1 mL/kg (0.01 mg/kg) every 5 min as necessary. Subcutaneous epinephrine will be less effective in the hypotensive patient, but may be necessary if there is no IV access. Antihistamines may exacerbate hypotension.

The treatment of pediatric contrast reactions follows similar algorithms to treatment plans for adult reactions. Drug dosages are weight dependent, and it is helpful to have a chart posted in each room where contrast is administered, listing pediatric emergency medications and weight-based dosages (Table 4.1).

Pediatric airway management

Children's airways are smaller in diameter and more easily compromised than the adult airway (Table 4.2). Children's necks are shorter, their tongues are relatively

Table 4.1 Pediatric dose schedules

Medication	Dose
Epinephrine	
SubQ (1:1000)	0.01 mL/kg (0.01 mg/kg), repeat in 15–30 min, max 0.3 mL/dose
IV (1:10000)	0.1 mL/kg (0.01 mg/kg), repeat every 5–15 min as necessary; give slowly and titrate to effect.
Atropine	0.02 mg/kg IV
	Minimum initial dose: 0.1 mg
	Maximum initial dose: 0.6 mg (infants and children)
	1.0 mg (adolescents)
	Maximum total dose (0.04 mg/kg): for example,
	1.0 mg (children)
	2.0 mg (adolescents)
Beta-2-agonist inhaler	2 puffs every 20–30 min, as necessary
Albuterol	(90–180 µg)
(Proventil®)	
(Ventolin®)	
Corticosteroids	
Methylprednisolone	2.0 mg/kg IV loading dose
(Solumedrol®)	
H-1 antihistamine:	
Diphenhydramine	1–2 mg/kg IV or PO, up to maximum dose of 50 mg
(Benadryl®)	
Diuretic	
Furosemide	1.0 mg/kg
(Lasix®)	Maximum total dose of 40 mg

Conversion: kilograms (kg) = pounds (lbs)/2.2

Table 4.2 Reasons for increased susceptibility to respiratory emergencies in infants and children

1 Obligatory nose breathing, higher metabolic requirements, inefficient immune system in young infants

2 Anatomical components of large tongue, small mandible and soft epiglottis

3 Smaller diameter of airways – easily occluded and collapsible, greater resistance to airflow

4 More compliant, unstable chest wall due to anatomical configuration of ribs, cartilage and diaphragm

5 Immature musculature – easy fatigability of diaphragm and poor control of upper airway patency

6 Behavioral immaturity – unable to verbalize distress; prone to foreign-body aspiration

larger, and there is more redundant soft tissue in the pharynx.[6] Inflammatory conditions of the upper and lower airway are common, and can further compromise a small airway (Fig. 4.1). Neck and mediastinal masses, such as lymphoma, abscess or cystic hygroma, may cause significant compression of the airway. Children with congenital anomalies of the head and neck, such as hypoplasia of the mandible (micrognathia), may be predisposed to airway compromise, especially when sedated. Aspiration may occlude the airway or impair oxygen exchange. The risk of aspiration is increased in sedated, critically ill or neurologically impaired children.

Managing the pediatric airway begins with correct head positioning.[7] Spontaneous ventilation may be improved with simple repositioning maneuvers. The recumbent child tends to lie with the upper airway in a flexed position due to prominence of the skull occiput relative to the shoulders. The airway position can be improved by placing a pad or towel under the child's shoulders, which elevates the upper torso and allows the neck to return to a neutral position. The chin lift and jaw thrust are useful methods for more urgent airway management (see illustrations in Chapter 5).

Suction is critical for clearing the upper airway and reducing the possibility of aspiration. Either mechanical or wall vacuum suction should be available and easy to use.

Pediatric respiratory emergency equipment should always be available. This includes high-flow oxygen and oxygen-delivery devices such as a simple face mask, partial nonrebreather mask, bag-valve mask, mouth-to-mask, and airway adjuncts such as oropharyngeal airways and intubation equipment. It is useful to have a separate box of pediatric-sized airway equipment attached to the emergency cart if both children and adults are cared for in the same area.

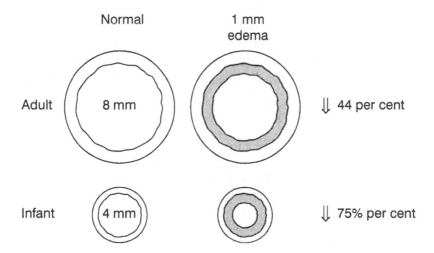

Figure 4.1 Illustration of the effect of reactive edema on the adult and pediatric airway. One millimeter of mucusal edema narrows the adult airway by about 44 per cent, whereas the same 1 mm of edema causes a 75 per cent decrease in the pediatric airway due to the smaller calliber of the child's airway relative to that of the adult.

For a child with spontaneous respiration or mild distress, a simple face mask delivers oxygen more effectively than a nasal cannula, and will deliver an oxygen concentration of 30–60 per cent at an oxygen flow rate of 6–10 L/min. This mask may be supported near the child's face to provide 'blow-by' oxygen if the child will not tolerate covering of the mouth and nose. The unrestrained conscious child in respiratory distress will want to sit in the position in which he or she is most comfortable, and allowing this may well facilitate care.

Moderate to severe respiratory distress in a spontaneously ventilating child may be more effectively treated with a partial nonrebreather mask. The partial nonrebreather mask has a reservoir bag for inspiration of high concentrations of oxygen, and side vents for expiration of exhaled gases. The reservoir bag should be fully inflated with oxygen when it is being correctly used. This system can deliver 90 per cent oxygen at 10–12 L/min.

Bag-valve-mask ventilation is reserved for the nonbreathing, unconscious child. It provides an effective means of oxygenation until the child can be transferred to an acute-care setting or until emergency respiratory personnel arrive to help manage the child and his or her airway. The correct-sized mask covers the face from the bridge of the nose to the cleft of the chin. The head should be in the neutral or chin-lift position, with a tight seal of the mask to the face with one or two hands. The bag should be connected to an inflated reservoir which has a constant oxygen source. Bag-valve-mask ventilation is most effectively performed by two people. One person holds the face mask with both hands in order to maintain a tight seal and optimal head position, while the second person ventilates by compressing the air bag (see illustrations in Chapter 5). Fingertip compression of the bag is used on infants. The ventilation rate varies with age (see Table 4.3). Bag-valve-mask ventilation may be more effective when used in conjunction with an oropharyngeal airway in the unconscious patient. The oropharyngeal airway assists in lifting the tongue off the back of the throat and directs oxygen past the oropharynx into the hypopharynx. The length of the oropharyngeal airway in a given child should match the distance from the side of the mouth to the angle of the mandible. The oropharyngeal airway should be inserted under direct visualization with the aid of a tongue depressor. The

Table 4.3 Normal vital signs by age

Age	Respiration rate (breaths/min)	Pulse rate (beats/min)
Newborn	30–60	100–160
1–6 weeks	30–60	100–160
6 months	25–40	90–140
1 year	20–40	90–130
3 years	20–30	80–120
6 years	12–25	70–110
10 years	12–20	60–90

oropharyngeal airway must be properly inserted or it can occlude the airway by pushing the tongue to the back of the throat.

An alternative to the bag-valve mask is mouth-to-mask ventilation with supplementary oxygen. Mouth-to-mask ventilation relies on a barrier valve to protect emergency personnel from contact with oral or gastric materials. This method also allows a single emergency worker to ventilate the patient effectively, since both hands are available to ensure a tight seal of the mask around the child's nose and mouth and to maintain optimal airway position. An oropharyngeal airway adjunct may also help to maintain the child's airway. Mouth-to mask ventilation may be difficult to maintain by a single emergency worker for an extended length of time.

Management of the airway in children in a situation of acute respiratory distress requires personnel who are aware of the unique features of the pediatric airway and trained in the use of medication and oxygen-delivery systems for children. The correct pediatric-sized airway equipment and medication should be readily available wherever children with the potential for airway compromise are cared for.

References

1. Cohen MD. Comparison of intravenous contrast agents for CT studies in children. *Acta Radiologica* 1992; **33**: 592–5.

2. Cohen MD. Intravenous use of ionic and nonionic contrast agents in children. *Radiology* 1994; **191**: 793–4.

3. Gooding CA, Berdon WE, Brodeur AE, Rowen M. Adverse reactions to intravenous pyelography in children. *American Journal of Roentgenology* 1975; **123**: 802–4.

4. Wood BP, Lane AT, Rabinowitz R. Cutaneous reaction to contrast material. *Radiology* 1988; **69**: 739–40.

5. Cohen MD. A review of the toxicity of nonionic contrast agents in children. *Investigative Radiology* 1993; **28** (Supplement 5): S87–S93.

6. Barkin RM, Rosen P. *Pediatric emergency medicine: concepts and clinical practice*, 2nd edn. St Louis, MO: Mosby Publishers, 1997.

7. Ludwig S, Kettrick RG. Resuscitation – pediatric basic and advanced life support. *Textbook of pediatric emergency care, 3rd edn*. Baltimore, MD: Williams and Wilkins, 1993.

5 Airways and oxygen for adult emergencies in the radiology department

Daniel G. Hankins and William H. Bush Jr

An airway must be established for every patient or they will die. Not only is the airway important, but it may be the most important aspect of all. The purpose of this chapter is to review airway structure and function, basic airway maneuvers, and modes of oxygen administration.

The upper airway and its evaluation

The semiconscious or unconscious patient usually has an airway problem because, when the upper airway relaxes in such a patient, the tongue becomes floppy and obstructs the airway (Fig. 5.1). You must perform an airway maneuver such as a *chin lift* or *modified jaw thrust* to help to open the airway (Figs 5.2a and b). Remember that an altered level of consciousness by definition means that an airway problem exists.

Although it would be unusual in the radiology suite, one must always remember that an aspirated foreign body with complete airway obstruction requires one or more abdominal thrusts (Heimlich maneuver) in the adult. An adult with a complete airway obstruction often shows the universal sign of airway distress, where the victim clutches his or her throat and cannot speak. On the other hand, an adult with only partial airway obstruction may be doing a good job of trying to clear the airway, but such a patient with incomplete airway obstruction may be moving air either well or poorly. If the patient is moving air well and attempting to clear the airway on his or her own, it is probably best to not intervene. In this scenario, your efforts may complicate matters by turning an incomplete airway obstruction into a complete one. However, if the patient is making poor efforts at ventilation and clearing the airway, you should intervene carefully.

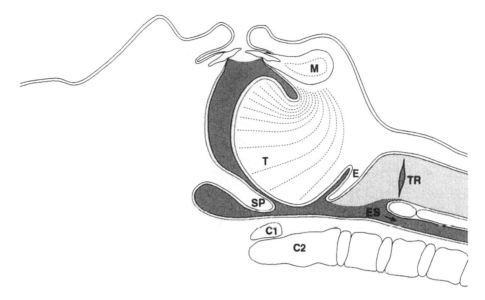

Figure 5.1 Sagittal section through the orohypopharynx of a comatose supine patient showing how the relaxed tongue drops downward and substantially occludes the airway (M = mandible; T = tongue; SP = soft palate and uvula; C1 and C2 = first two cervical vertebrae; E = epiglottis; ES = esophagus; TR = trachea).

The Heimlich maneuver is performed by forcefully applying thrust in the epigastric area below the rib-cage and xiphoid and above the navel. In the patient who is awake, it is performed from behind with the patient standing or sitting. If the patient is unconscious, the abdominal thrusts are made with the patient supine. A finger-sweep of the mouth may also be attempted in an unconscious patient as part of the sequence, as noted below.

The American Heart Association recommends the following procedure for a choking patient who becomes unconscious.[1]

1 If a syncopal episode is witnessed and a foreign body is suspected, the emergency worker should open the mouth of the unconscious patient and perform the 'finger-sweep.'

2 If the patient is found unconscious or no foreign body is suspected during witnessed loss of consciousness, rescue breathing should be attempted.

3 If the patient cannot be ventilated even after attempts to reposition the jaw and airway, the Heimlich maneuver should be performed (up to five times). The patient's mouth should then be opened and a finger-sweep performed. Finally, ventilation should be attempted.

4 The sequence of Heimlich maneuver, finger-sweep, and attempt to ventilate should be repeated.

5 These efforts should be repeated and continued as long as necessary.

(a)

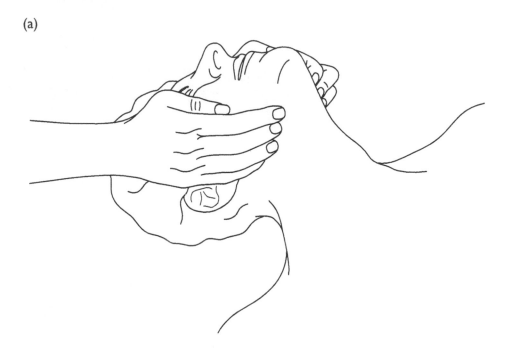

(b)

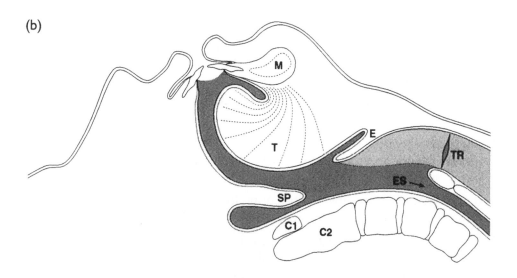

Figure 5.2 The chin lift or jaw thrust maneuver (a) with upward positioning of the mandible elevates the tongue from the posterior orohypopharynx (b) and re-establishes an adequate airway (compare with Figure 5.1).

In the setting of radiologic interventions, upper airway obstruction may be due to laryngeal edema or, rarely, to laryngeal spasm. In these cases, mechanical intervention may *not* be of help. However, airway positioning should always be tried. In the case of laryngeal problems, pharmacologic intervention with epinephrine will be necessary (see Chapter 3 on treatment of contrast reactions). In the worst-case scenario, a surgical airway should be considered (see below).

Airway adjuncts

In addition to airway positioning, there are several artificial airway adjuncts that may be helpful.

Suctioning

A patient who is in difficulty almost always empties his or her stomach. Bulk material needs to be cleared from the mouth or oropharynx with a finger, a tonsil sucker, or one of the newer self-contained suction devices, such as the V-Vac. Liquid or smaller particulate matter can be cleared with the traditional tube suction. Proper suctioning after the initial oral clearing involves the following procedure.

1 Oxygenate for 3 min or so before suctioning;

2 Make sure that suction is on and working;

3 Suction after you are in the oropharynx and while withdrawing, not on entering;

4 Suction for only 15 seconds (5 seconds if assisting ventilations), unless more gross material is present;

5 Start high-flow oxygen again immediately post suctioning.

Oral airway (or oropharyngeal airway)

This device is the usual airway adjunct, short of intubation (Fig. 5.3). In adults, the appropriate size is selected by measuring from the angle of the mouth to the angle of the mandible. Usually, in an adult, the size will be around a #7 or #8. The airway is then inserted upside down and rotated through 180° in an adult. There are also pediatric-sized oral airways, which are not inserted by rotation as in adults, but with the assistance of a tongue blade. Because they will irritate the gag reflex, oral airways are better tolerated in more lethargic patients.

Nasopharyngeal airway

This airway is often called the 'trumpet' airway because of its flared end at the nose. This is an ideal airway for patients with clenched teeth or who are semiconscious and will not tolerate an oral airway because of their gag reflex. An appropriate size is chosen, based on the diameter of the nares and the distance from the nose to the angle of the jaw. The well-lubricated tube is inserted into the nose up to the flared end. In general, this is a device for use in adults.

(a)

(b)

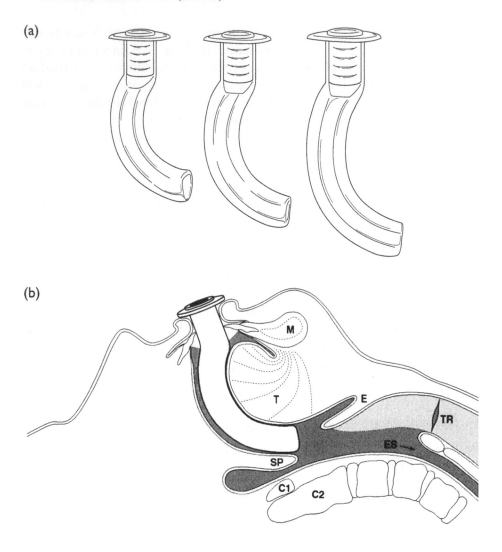

Figure 5.3   The oral airway. (a) Three sizes are illustrated. (b) This is the usual airway adjunct for maintaining an elevated position of the tongue so that an adequate airway exists.

Both nasal and oral airways are useful in conjuction with a bag-valve mask (B-V-M) if that mode of assisted ventilation is deemed necessary.

Endotracheal intubation

This is the 'gold standard' of airway management. However, it requires skill and experience.[2] The best option for the occasional intubator is to try once but then to use a nasal or oral airway with bag-valve-mask (B-V-M) ventilation. *If you have not performed intubation for a long time, do not try now.* Instead, put all your efforts into achieving good B-V-M ventilation for the patient. One pitfall of ventilating with B-V-M consists of not obtaining an adequate tidal volume because of poor mask seal. One person may find it very difficult to obtain a good seal with one hand on the mask while ventilating the patient with the other hand. For neophytes at ventilatory assistance, it is better to make it a two-person job. One person holds the mask on for a good seal, while the second person squeezes the ambu or anesthesia bag to get an adequate tidal volume (Fig. 5.4).

For endotracheal intubation, the proper tube size is selected (usually 6.5–7.5 mm for women and 7.5–8.5 mm for men). The balloon is checked with 10 mL of air, and the tube is lubricated. The laryngoscope, with either a straight or curved blade (depending on personal preference) is checked and inserted. The vocal cords are visualized and the tube is placed. This is not as easy as it sounds, particularly for the inexperienced. Non-operating-room intubations can be difficult in even the most experienced hands.

One hint for successful intubation is to pretend that you are using the laryngoscope to lift the head via the mandible (obviously this applies to patients for whom you are not concerned about their cervical spine status!). This will give you the

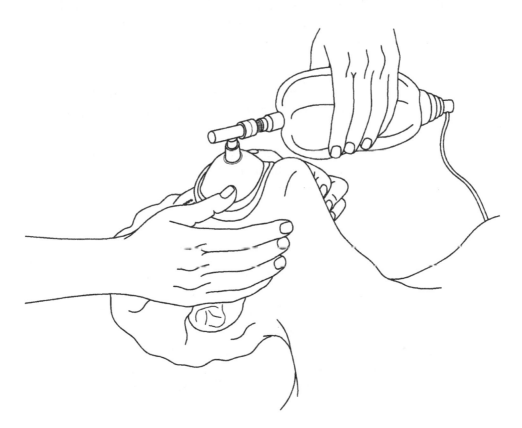

Figure 5.4 Ventilation with a bag-valve mask is recommended for initial ventilation of the patient, particularly for an operator not experienced in endotracheal intubation. Although it can be achieved by one person, maintenance of a proper seal about the month is usually better accomplished when two people team together to provide the seal and ventilation.

right direction of force to visualize the vocal cords. The other main point is to ventilate the patient for several minutes with a B-V-M before attempting to intubate. Pre-oxygenation will give you more time to intubate.

As a last resort, a surgical airway may be required. Classical cricothyroidotomy may not be the best method to use, but a needle cricothyrostomy can buy some time for the patient. A needle through the cricothyroid membrane can be ventilated successfully with jet insufflation, which can be rigged up with simple oxygen tubing from wall oxygen.

Oxygen

Be aggressive with oxygen, which is a very powerful and important drug. The patient is potentially very ill and therefore needs 'serious' and not 'courtesy' oxygen. A nasal cannula only offers an FiO_2 of 0.23–0.45 at best (room air = 0.21; 100 per cent O_2 = 1.0). There are many mask options available, but for 'serious' oxygen use a partial non-rebreather mask at 12–15 L/min of oxygen flow. Pulse oximetry should be available, as it is a cheap, non-invasive, easy-to-use method of monitoring oxygen saturation in a patient's blood. Pulse oximeters are recommended in areas where a patient can suddenly deteriorate.

Summary

- In any serious situation, the paramount problem is maintenance of airway and ventilation with supplemental oxygen to maintain pO_2, pCO_2 and pH within physiologic ranges.

- If an airway is not established, the patient will die no matter what else is done. Every effort must be made to establish an airway and to ventilate the patient before moving on to other measures.

References

1   American Heart Association. Adult advanced cardiac life support. In Guidelines for cardiopulmonary resuscitation and emergency cardiac care: recommendations of the 1992 Conference. *Journal of the American Medical Association* 1992; **268**: 2199–204.

2   Danzl DF. Advanced airway support. In: Tintinalli JE, Krome RL, Ruiz E, eds. *Emergency medicine: a comprehensive study guide. American College of Emergency Physicians*, 4th edn. New York: McGraw-Hill, 1996: 39–49.

Cardiac dysrhythmia management in the radiology department

Geoffrey S. Ferguson

6

As radiologists assume pivotal roles in increasingly complex and occasionally hazardous procedures, they must also accept the clinical responsibility for both successful and adverse outcomes. This philosophy is shared by the Society of Cardiovascular and Interventional Radiology: 'The radiologist cannot rely on others to recognize and manage the problems that arise in his or her patient's care.'[1] While the majority of these events will be minor, many will be significant and some even life threatening. There is significant comorbidity in some radiology patient populations, particularly those with cardiovascular and pulmonary disease. In a study of factors that influence long-term percutaneous transluminal angioplasty (PTA) success,[2] Capek found that at the time of presentation for femoral-popliteal PTA, 50 per cent of patients were hypertensive, 90 per cent smoked more than one pack per day, 33 per cent were diabetic and 18 per cent showed evidence of generalized cardiovascular disease. In patients presenting with intermittent claudication, Hertzer[3] found that 27 per cent had severe coronary artery disease (CAD), as did 29 per cent of those presenting with rest pain or gangrene.[3] In addition, some procedures are performed on critically ill patients, e.g. transjugular intrahepatic porto-systemic (TIPS) shunt, bronchial arterial embolization, inferior vena cava (IVC) filters and pulmonary angiography. Thus it becomes increasingly important for radiologists to become familiar not only with the specific complications that may be encountered during procedures, but with some basic principles concerning the recognition and treatment of other acute adverse events. The importance of early recognition and treatment of pre hospital sudden cardiac arrest and an integrated 'chain of survival' concept has significantly improved survival rates in out-of-hospital cardiac arrest,[4-9] and many of these principles can be applied to radiology departments. This chapter deals with aspects of recognition and management of cardiac dysrhythmias. For acquisition of cardiac resuscitative skills, the practitioner is urged to complete the American Heart Association's Advanced Cardiac Life Support (ACLS) course.

Dysrhythmia origins

Cardiac dysrhythmias can be thought of as disturbances of impulse formation (disturbed automaticity), alterations of conduction, or combinations of both.[10] Examples of disturbed automaticity might include acceleration or deceleration of the sinoatrial (SA) node (sinus tachycardia, sinus bradycardia), as well as impulses arising from ectopic foci. Examples of the latter would include premature beats in the atria, atrioventricular (AV) junction or ventricles. Atrial and ventricular tachycardias can also be regarded as disturbances of automaticity, with rapid firing of an ectopic pacemaker focus as the underlying mechanism. Conduction disturbances can be seen with slowed conduction, especially through the AV node, where varying degrees of atrioventricular block occur. Re-entry can also be viewed as an alteration of conduction, but on a more local level. Atrial flutter with 3:1 block and premature atrial contraction with first-degree AV block are examples of combined alterations of automaticity and conduction.

Electrocardiogram (ECG)

The electrocardiogram records the complex electrical events that occur in the heart with each cardiac cycle by assuming that the body can be regarded as a giant conductor of electrical currents. Any two points on the body surface can be connected to positive and negative 'leads,' with current flowing towards the positive electrode producing an upward deflection on the ECG trace. The 12-lead ECG 'looks' at the electrical activity in 12 different directions, any one of which could be used to evaluate the rhythm. The 'standard limb-leads' are conveniently selectable on most cardiac monitors by using only three leads connected to the patient. By convention, the resulting complexes are labeled the P wave, the QRS complex and the T wave. (see Fig. 6.1). Atrial depolarization produces the P wave, which is normally upright in lead II. The PR interval represents the normally slower conduction through the AV node, and should not exceed 0.2 s. The QRS complex represents ventricular depolarization, with the Q wave (the first negative deflection) not always visible. As viewed in lead II, the R wave is the next positive (upward) deflection, followed by a negative S wave. Because ventricular depolarization is a rapid event, the normal QRS is narrow and should not exceed 0.1 s. Atrial repolarization is obscured by the QRS complex. The ST segment represents the time from complete depolarization of the ventricles to the beginning of repolarization. Since no net electrical activity is occurring during this recovery phase of the cardiac cycle, the ST segment is normally flat. With ischemia or injury, the ST segment may be elevated or depressed. Ventricular repolarization results in the T wave, which is usually upright in lead II.

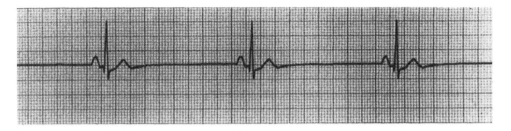

Figure 6.1 Sinus bradycardia.

Basic rhythm strip interpretation

Two basic questions need to be answered when performing dysrhythmia interpretation.

1 What is the rate?

2 What is the rhythm?

Rate determination will be considered first.

By convention, the ECG paper runs at a rate of 25 mm/s, resulting in each small box representing 0.04 s and each large box 0.20 s.[10,11] There are many methods for rate determination. One method is to divide the number of large boxes of an R-R interval into 300. An aid to this approach is to memorize the descending '300–150–100–75–60–50' sequence. Rates that fall between these values can be interpolated. A faster but less accurate method involves simply counting the number of R waves in 6 s (there are 1 s 'tick marks' at the top of the strip) and multiply by 10.

Once the rate has been determined, rhythm analysis begins by assessing regularity. This is usually apparent from visual inspection, but in borderline cases the measurement of successive R-R intervals with calipers or paper and sharp pencil may be required. To analyze the P waves, one should remember that the normal P wave is upright in lead II, and all of the P waves should look identical. If the P waves vary in their morphology, the impulses are arising from different locations within the atria. The next step is to analyze the relationship between the P waves and the QRS complexes, which should be one to one. Each QRS complex should be preceded by a P wave, and the PR interval should be constant and less than 0.20 s (one big box). Finally, the QRS complex should be narrow: 0.11 s is borderline, and 0.12 s (three small boxes) is prolonged. This is an important determination, because with a QRS of normal duration, the impulse must originate above the bundle of His (SA node, atria or AV junction). With a wide (prolonged by > 0.12 s) QRS, impulse formation is either in the ventricles or there is altered ventricular conduction of a supraventricular impulse.

Sinus and atrial dysrhythmias

The aim of this section is to summarize some of the major features of commonly encountered sinus and atrial dysrhythmias.[7,10–16] The following rhythms will be covered in this section:

- sinus bradycardia;
- sinus tachycardia;
- paroxysmal supraventricular tachycardia (PSVT);
- multifocal atrial tachycardia (MAT);
- premature atrial contraction (PAC);
- atrial flutter;
- atrial fibrillation.

Sinus bradycardia (Fig. 6.1)

Etiology
Slowing of the sinus node from intrinsic nodal disease (e.g. ischemia), increased parasympathetic tone (pain, anxiety), athletic conditioning, medication (e.g. propranolol, digitalis).

Identifying characteristics
The rate is less than 60 beats/min, but usually greater than 40 beats/min. Both atrial and ventricular rhythms are regular, and P waves are normal. The PR interval is normal or slightly prolonged. The QRS complex is normal, as is conduction.

Risk
Because of decreased cardiac output, syncope and angina may occur. Junctional or ventricular escape beats may occur.

Precautions
Avoid negative chronotropic agents such as propranolol and digitalis. Maintain blood pressure (volume expansion, Trendelenberg). Be alert for premature ventricular contractions (PVCs).

Treatment
No treatment may be required if the patient is asymptomatic. If there is hypotension, angina, ventricular escape beats, or rate less than 30 beats/min, IV atropine is the treatment of choice. If unsuccessful, chronotropic support with dopamine, epinephrine or isoproterenol may be necessary. Under extreme circumstances, a pacemaker may be needed.

Sinus tachycardia (Fig. 6.2)

Etiology
Accelerated firing of the sinus node, with a multitude of causes, including pain, anxiety, fever, hypovolemia, exertion, medication (e.g. epinephrine), hypoxia, or a need for increased cardiac output.

Identifying characteristics
The rate is usually 100–160 beats/min. Atrial and ventricular rates are regular. The P wave is normal, but may be difficult to find because of the rapid rate; it may be superimposed on the T wave. The PR interval may be at the lower limits of normal. The QRS is normal, as is conduction.

Risk
The increased rate may precipitate cardiac decompensation in patients with borderline cardiac function. Myocardial oxygen consumption may rise high enough to unmask angina, particularly with underlying coronary artery disease.

Precautions
Observe for signs of left ventricular failure (orthopnea, cough, dyspnea, restlessness). Minimize anxiety if possible.

Treatment
Treat the underlying cause.

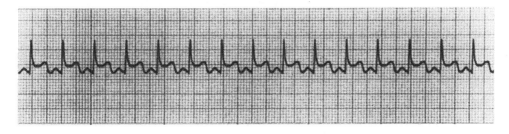

Figure 6.2 Sinus tachycardia; also, S-T segment elevation present.

Paroxysmal supraventricular tachycardia (PSVT) (Fig. 6.3)

Etiology
PSVT should be distinguished from the more generic term 'supraventricular tachycardia', which includes any tachycardia due to rapid impulse formation above the level of the AV node (sinus tachycardia, paroxysmal atrial tachycardia (PAT), atrial flutter, atrial fibrillation). 'Paroxysmal' is the key word. Two forms of PSVT are recognized, namely AV nodal re-entrant tachycardia, and orthodromic

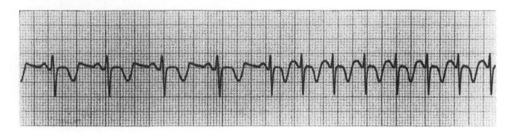

Figure 6.3 Paroxysmal supraventricular tachycardia (PSVT).

AV re-entrant tachycardia. See the article by Caruso for a complete discussion of differentiating between the two major forms of PSVT.[17]

Identifying characteristics
Three key features characterize PSVT.

1 It starts abruptly.

2 It ends abruptly.

3 There is 1:1 conduction – the ventricles respond to every impulse generated by the supraventricular focus.

The rate is usually 150–250 beats/min, both atrial and ventricular. The rhythm is perfectly regular. P waves are present, but may be very difficult to identify, and may not have the normal rounded shape, since they do not originate in the SA node. If a PR interval can be measured, it is usually within normal limits. The QRS complex is normal, except in the presence of an accessory pathway.

Risk
An uncontrolled rapid ventricular rate may lead to myocardial ischemia and, eventually, to cardiac decompensation.

Precautions
As with sinus tachycardia, observe for signs of cardiac decompensation or myocardial ischemia. Provide oxygen as necessary.

Treatment
Vagal stimulation such as coughing, unilateral carotid sinus massage and the Valsalva maneuver are simple and often effective measures.[18] Adenosine is a highly effective IV medication for terminating PSVT, although its effect is short-lived, and it may also transiently increase the degree of AV block sufficiently to uncover underlying atrial activity.[15] IV verapamil is also effective, but should not be given to patients with wide complex tachycardias.[17,19] If the patient becomes symptomatic (e.g. with angina, diaphoresis, hypotension), synchronized cardioversion should be used immediately with energy levels of 100 joules. This almost always terminates the tachycardia.[20]

Multifocal atrial tachycardia

Etiology
This rhythm is most commonly seen in hypoxic patients with chronic obstructive pulmonary disease.[11,18] Atrial foci from multiple different sites initiate impulse formation, resulting in an irregularly irregular rhythm that resembles atrial fibrillation in this regard. A high index of suspicion in a clinical setting of chronic obstructive pulmonary disease (COPD) may help in the diagnosis.

Identifying characteristics
The atrial and ventricular rates are 100–180 beats/min.[18] The rhythm is irregularly irregular. P waves are present, but vary in morphology, and the PR interval is variable. The QRS complex is normal. This rhythm is most often seen in patients who have COPD.

Risk
The main problem with this rhythm is confusing it with atrial fibrillation and treating it as such with digitalis, to which it is notoriously resistant.

Precautions
In a setting of COPD, examine the rhythm strip carefully in multiple leads for evidence of multiformed P waves. Evaluate the patient for clinical signs of hypoxia.

Treatment
Treatment of this rhythm is directed at correcting the underlying hypoxia and any associated metabolic abnormalities.

Premature atrial contraction (PAC) (Fig. 6.4)

Etiology
This single-beat dysrhythmia is the result of spontaneous depolarization of a temporary pacemaker focus somewhere in the atria other than the SA node. For the beat on which it occurs, it precludes firing of the SA node because it fires before

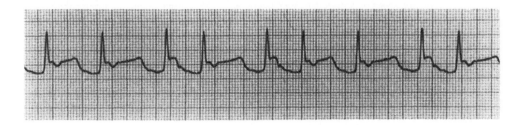

Figure 6.4 Premature atrial contraction (PAC).

the SA node's next expected beat, hence the term 'premature'. PAC's may occur without apparent cause, although they are associated with a number of factors, including caffeine, sympathomimetic medications, alcohol, hypoxia and elevation of atrial pressure.

Identifying characteristics

The underlying rate is usually normal (60–100 beats/min), but PACs may occur with any sinus rate. The rhythm is momentarily irregular due to the early firing of the atrial focus. Because the PAC depolarizes the SA node along with the rest of the atria, the SA node begins the generation of another impulse later than it normally would, due to the extra conduction time from the ectopic atrial focus to the SA node. Thus the next normal sinus beat (P) occurs after a brief 'noncompensatory' pause. The premature (P') wave will have a different shape to the P waves of the sinus beats because of its abnormal location. The P'R interval is variable but often prolonged. The QRS complex is normal unless there is aberrant ventricular conduction. There may also be variable AV block of the premature beat.

Risk

There is no significant risk from occasional PACs. If they are frequent (> 8/min), there may be an increased likelihood of atrial flutter or fibrillation.

Precautions

If anxiety is present, reassurance is needed. Monitor the frequency of PACs.

Treatment

Correction of the underlying cause (removal of caffeine, sympathomimetic medications, etc.) is the mainstay of treatment.

Atrial flutter (Fig. 6.5)

Etiology

An atrial focus, probably the result of re-entry at the atrial level, supersedes the SA node because of its faster rate. This rhythm may be seen in association with mitral or tricuspid valvular heart disease, coronary artery disease or cor pulmonale.

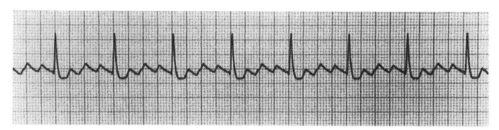

Figure 6.5   Atrial flutter.

Identifying characteristics

The atrial rate is rapid, usually 250–350 beats/min. The atrial rhythm is regular. The ventricular rhythm varies with the number of impulses transmitted through the AV node. The P waves resemble a 'picket-fence,' or 'sawtooth' in lead II, often referred to as 'flutter waves.' At slower rates (e.g. an atrial rate of 220 beats/min), it is possible to have 1:1 conduction, but most often there is a physiologic second-degree block at the AV node, resulting in 2:1 or 3:1 conduction.[10] The QRS is normal.

Risk

Severe hemodynamic compromise may occur within minutes with 1:1 conduction and rapid ventricular rates. Cardiac output can fall dramatically because of insufficient filling time. Even if systemic perfusion is adequate, there may be severe demands on myocardial oxygen consumption, and angina or left ventricular failure may ensue.

Precautions

Monitor the ECG for ventricular rate. Observe for clinical signs of hemodynamic compromise.

Treatment

With 3:1 or 4:1 conduction, ventricular rates may be slow enough for treatment to be unnecessary. For fast ventricular rates with hemodynamic compromise, synchronized cardioversion at low energy (25–50 joules) is the therapy of choice.[10,18] For rapid rates without hemodynamic compromise, calcium-channel blockers and beta-blockers can be used.

Atrial fibrillation (AF) (Fig. 6.6)

Etiology

Possibly the result of multiple ectopic foci or multiple areas of atrial re-entry, this rhythm produces a chaotic atrial electrical and mechanical process, with no organized atrial contraction. There is usually underlying organic heart disease.

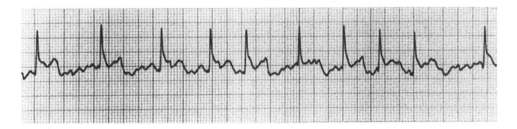

Figure 6.6   Atrial fibrillation.

Identifying characteristics

The atrial rate cannot be measured, and there are no P waves. The ventricular rate is variable, indeed random. The ventricular rhythm is described as irregularly irregular. There is a physiologic block of variable degree in the AV node. Some of the atrial impulses are conducted into but not through the AV node, where they depolarize the node and contribute to its overall refractoriness. Thus ventricular rates with AF are often lower than those seen with PSVT or atrial flutter.[10] The QRS is normal unless there is associated aberrant conduction.

Risk

With uncontrolled fast ventricular rates there is the potential for hemodynamic compromise, angina, pulmonary edema and cardiogenic shock. Atrial thrombi may form, with the risk of systemic embolization.

Precautions

Observe for clinical evidence of hemodynamic compromise or angina.

Treatment

If chronic atrial fibrillation is present and the patient is asymptomatic with no hemodynamic compromise, and the ventricular rate is 50–100 beats/min, no therapy may be required. For acute-onset AF with hemodynamic compromise, the therapy of choice is synchronized cardioversion at 100, 200, 300 and 360 joules. As with atrial flutter, rapid ventricular rates without hemodynamic compromise may be slowed with beta-blockers or calcium-channel blockers.[7] If AF with rapid ventricular response deteriorates to hemodynamic compromise within the first 72 h of onset, synchronized cardioversion may be required to slow the ventricular rate. After 72 h, there may be potential for increased risk of systemic embolization due to atrial thrombus formation.[10,11]

Conduction defects and ventricular dysrhythmias

The major dysrhythmias originating above the AV node have been described above. This section will discuss abnormal rhythms that are associated with altered conduction through the AV node, and those of ventricular origin.[7,10–16]

First-degree AV block (Fig. 6.7)

Etiology

This is simply delayed conduction through the AV node. It may be due to medication (especially digitalis, quinidine and procainamide), nodal injury as might occur in infarction, or nodal ischemia.

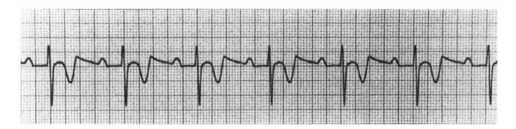

Figure 6.7 First-degree atrioventricular (AV) block.

Identifying characteristics
The rate is normal. The rhythm is regular and P waves are normal. The PR interval is prolonged to > 0.2 s (one big box). Conduction is otherwise normal, and the QRS complex is normal.

Risk
No particular risk is associated with this rhythm.

Precautions
In a setting of myocardial infarction, monitor for possible progression to second- or third-degree AV block.

Treatment
First-degree block of > 0.26 s may be treated with atropine to increase AV nodal conduction.

Second-degree AV block, type I (Fig. 6.8)

Note: this is sometimes called Mobitz I or Wenckebach.

Etiology
With AV nodal injury or ischemia it becomes progressively more difficult for succeeding impulses to pass through the node, until a beat is blocked entirely. This may also be seen in association with increased parasympathetic tone and medications such as propranolol and digoxin.

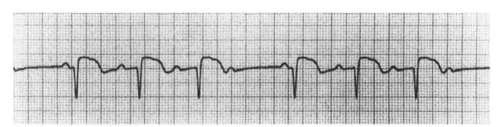

Figure 6.8 Second-degree AV block, type I.

Identifying characteristics

The atrial rate may be normal. The ventricular rate is slower than the atrial rate because of the blocked beats. The atrial rhythm is regular, while the ventricular rhythm is irregular. P waves are normal. The PR interval becomes progressively prolonged with a decreasing RR interval until a P wave is not conducted.[10,11] Usually only a single impulse is blocked, and the cycle is then repeated. As a result there is 'group beating', characterized by QRS complexes (and hopefully peripheral pulses) that come in groups until one is lost. The QRS is normal.

Risk

As a rule, the outlook is good, this often being a transient dysrhythmia following myocardial infarction. It should be considered potentially dangerous in that there may be progression to third-degree block (see below).

Precautions

Monitor for progression to third-degree block.

Treatment

Usually no therapy is needed. If the ventricular rate becomes excessively slow, and the patient is symptomatic as a result of this, atropine may be used.

Second-degree AV block, type II (Fig. 6.9)

Note: an alternative term for this is Mobitz II.

Etiology

This block is associated with an organic lesion (e.g. infarct, ischemia) just below the AV node, either in the bundle of His or a bundle branch. Unlike type I second-degree block, it is not due to medication or increased parasympathetic tone. One or more impulses are not conducted through the lesion, resulting in dropped beats.

Identifying characteristics

The atrial rate may be normal. The ventricular rate depends on the frequency of the block. The atrial rhythm is regular, but the ventricular rhythm is irregular. The

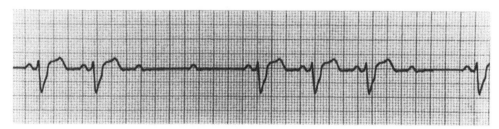

Figure 6.9 Second-degree AV block, type II.

P waves are normal. Unlike type I block, the PR interval does not lengthen prior to a dropped beat.[10,11] Non-conducted beats may be random, or with 2:1, 3:1, or 4:1 conduction ratios. If the block is occurring in the bundle of His, the QRS complex will be normal. More often the block is in one of the bundle branches, and as a result the usual type II block is associated with a widened QRS complex.

Risk
Unlike type I second-degree block, this rhythm represents a significant risk because of its propensity to deteriorate unpredictably to third-degree (complete) heart block.[10] This is especially common in a setting of acute myocardial infarction.

Precautions
Monitor closely for widening of the QRS complex and third-degree block. The wider the QRS, the lower in the conduction system is the block, and further prolongation of the QRS may herald complete heart block. Since a temporary or permanent pacemaker is indicated for this rhythm, preparation for pacing would be prudent.

Treatment
Frequently there will be a need for temporary pacing while preparations are made for insertion of a permanent pacemaker. Atropine or isoproterenol may be required as temporary measures, but a pacemaker is the treatment of choice.

Third-degree (complete) AV block (Fig. 6.10)

Etiology
There is a complete absence of conduction at the level of the AV node, bundle of His or bundle branch. If it is at the AV node, the block may be due to increased parasympathetic tone, medication or infarction/ischemia, but if it is below the AV node the block is most often due to infarction or ischemia, and usually involves both right and left bundle branches.[10] If the block is at the AV node, a junctional pacemaker focus will usually be present, with a rate of 40–60 beats/min, and the prognosis is more favorable. Infranodal third-degree block will usually result in a ventricular escape focus, but immediate pacing is still likely to be needed.

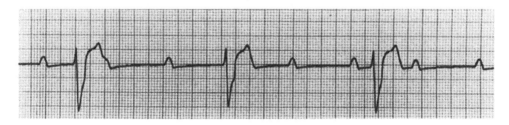

Figure 6.10   Third-degree (complete) AV block.

Identifying characteristics

The atrial rate is faster than the ventricular rate. The rhythm is regular for both atrial and ventricular foci, but they are totally independent of each other. The P waves may be normal. The PR interval is random because of the lack of association between atrial and ventricular rhythms (there is no AV conduction). If the block is at the AV node, the QRS will be normal, indicating the presence of a junctional escape rhythm, usually at 40–60 beats/min. For infranodal third-degree block the QRS will be widened, particularly at the bundle-branch level.

Risk

If the block is at the AV node and there is a junctional rhythm at a rate sufficient to maintain cardiac output, there may be adequate perfusion. For infranodal complete heart block there will probably be hemodynamic compromise. Even with a ventricular escape focus this is not a stable rhythm, and there is a propensity to develop ventricular fibrillation or asystole.

Precautions

Monitor the ECG for block at a lower level in the conduction system, ventricular fibrillation or asystole. Provide oxygen, and begin preparations for pacemaker insertion.

Treatment

For block at the AV node with a ventricular rate that is too slow to maintain adequate cardiac output, atropine is the drug of choice, with temporary pacemaker insertion if atropine fails. For infranodal block a pacemaker is indicated. The patient's condition may require isoproterenol for chronotropic support prior to pacing.

Premature ventricular contraction (PVC) (Fig. 6.11)

Etiology

An irritable focus in the ventricle initiates an impulse before the next normally conducted beat. This may be seen in a variety of clinical situations, including hypoxia, acidosis, bradycardia, electrolyte imbalance, drug toxicity and myocardial infarction.[10]

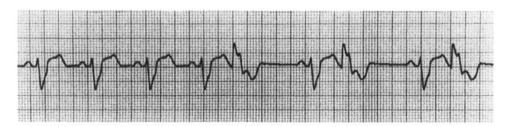

Figure 6.11 Premature ventricular contraction (PVC).

Identifying characteristics

The atrial and ventricular rates may be normal. The ventricular rhythm is irregular. P waves are not associated with the PVC complex unless there is retrograde atrial depolarization. The PR interval does not apply to the PVC. The QRS complex is wide and bizarre. Usually, there is a compensatory pause equal to two R-R intervals following the normal beat prior to the PVC, because the sinus-node impulse and PVC impulse tend to meet at the AV node, where neither can spread further because of the refractory period of the other.[10,11] Exceptions occur when the PVC falls between two normal sinus beats (interpolated PVC), resulting in no pause, and when the PVC reaches the atria and depolarizes the AV node prior to its next spontaneous impulse, resulting in a noncompensatory pause of less than two R-R intervals. The coupling interval (the time between the previous normal beat and the PVC) tends to be constant for ventricular beats arising from the same ectopic focus, and their morphology is the same (unifocal PVCs). For ventricular beats arising from more than one focus, or from the same focus and with varying conduction, the coupling interval and QRS morphology will vary (multifocal or multiformed PVCs). By definition, three or more PVCs in succession are termed ventricular tachycardia. PVCs occurring on every other beat are termed bigeminy, and those occurring on every third beat are referred to as trigeminy.

Risk

Although it has been taught that six or more PVCs per minute and PVCs falling on a T wave may be harbingers of ventricular tachycardia or fibrillation, the clinical setting in which the PVCs are occurring is probably a more important factor in risk assessment. PVCs of increasing frequency and the development of multifocal PVCs suggest increasing ventricular irritability, which in a clinical setting of acute myocardial infarction may have a different implication to, for example, a COPD patient with respiratory acidosis from carbon dioxide retention.

Precautions

Monitor for increasing frequency of PVCs, or multiformed PVCs. Depending on the clinical circumstances, consider preparing for lidocaine bolus and drip.

Treatment

Occasional PVCs in the asymptomatic patient without suspected heart disease do not require therapy. If the clinical situation indicates prompt treatment, IV lidocaine is the drug of choice, with procainamide for resistant cases.[10,11]

Ventricular tachycardia (VT) (Fig. 6.12)

Etiology

A commonly cited cause of VT is a local focus of re-entry, often due to a left ventricular scar from a previous infarction,[18,21] which sets up a 'circus' movement of

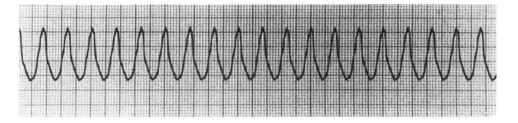

Figure 6.12 Ventricular tachycardia.

electrical current around the anatomic defect. This results in rhythmic impulse formation, conducted through the ventricles with variable effectiveness of contraction. Some VT will be slow enough to allow adequate time for ventricular filling, and if there is sufficiently organized ventricular mechanical activity, stroke volume may be sufficient to generate a pulse. However, there is often a precipitous fall in cardiac output.[10] VT is associated with multiple conditions, including coronary artery disease, dilated or hypertrophic cardiomyopathy, hypoxia, acidosis and electrolyte imbalance. Non-sustained VT may occur in as many as 50 per cent of all patients with congestive heart failure.[22] Despite its association with the above factors, the prognosis for surviving cardiac arrest is best when the underlying mechanism is VT, most commonly seen during in-hospital arrests.[15]

Identifying characteristics
The rate is greater than 100, usually 120–220 beats/min. The rhythm is regular. With slow enough ventricular rates , P waves may be visible, but because the AV node is being repeatedly depolarized by the ventricular impulses, there is complete AV dissociation. At faster rates, P waves are not visible. The PR interval does not apply. The QRS is wide and bizarre. There is no normal conduction, with an ectopic ventricular focus initiating impulse formation. Verapamil should not be administered as a diagnostic tool in wide complex tachycardia.[18]

Risk
There are multiple risks associated with sustained VT. Even if the patient has a pulse and is hemodynamically stable, myocardial oxygen consumption is greatly increased and there is a risk of deterioration to ventricular fibrillation. If there is a pulse but insufficient cardiac output for tissue perfusion, cardiogenic shock will ensue. Pulseless VT is not of course a perfusing rhythm.

Precautions
If the patient is conscious and breathing, 'cough version' may be employed if the onset of VT is witnessed. The patient is instructed to 'cough hard and keep coughing!'[10] Oxygen should be administered if the patient is breathing. Preparations for lidocaine administration and synchronized cardioversion or defibrillation should begin immediately.

Treatment

For hemodynamically stable VT with a palpable pulse, IV lidocaine is the drug of choice, followed by procainamide and bretylium. Patients who become hemodynamically unstable during the course of observation should receive synchronized cardioversion at 100–200 joules. Pulseless VT is treated with defibrillation, using the same procedure as for ventricular fibrillation (see section on resuscitation algorithms later in this chapter).

Ventricular fibrillation (VF) (Fig. 6.13)

Etiology

There is a total lack of organized cardiac electrical activity, with random, chaotic electrical currents in the ventricles, and no ventricular contraction. As a result there is no cardiac output. This is said to be the most common mechanism of cardiac arrest resulting from myocardial ischemia or infarction.[11]

Identifying characteristics

The rate is too chaotic to count. There really is no rhythm, but it could be described as irregular (indeed random). There are, of course, no P waves, QRS complexes or T waves.

Risk

If left untreated, this is a fatal rhythm.

Precautions

Check that it is VF and not artifact (i.e. check lead placements, lead selection, paddle placement and selection, etc.).

Treatment

Immediate defibrillation is the treatment of choice. Cardiopulmonary resuscitation (CPR) should be started, but should not delay defibrillation. If the first series of three shocks is unsuccessful, the patient is intubated and IV access is established. Liberal use of epinephrine in conjunction with continued CPR[10,15,23] and

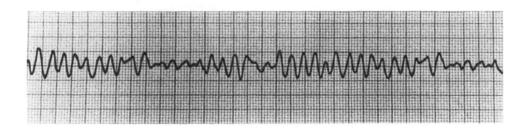

Figure 6.13   Ventricular fibrillation.

repeated attempts at defibrillation are justified. Lidocaine may also be administered (see section on resuscitation algorithms).

Defibrillation

Rapid defibrillation is the single most effective treatment for the patient in ventricular fibrillation,[7,10,11] and 'the sooner a patient in ventricular fibrillation can be defibrillated, the better the chance of survival.'[15] The aim of this section is to review the basic principles and procedures relating to defibrillation. Basic life support (BLS or basic CPR) will not be covered. For a complete review, the practitioner is urged to complete an ACLS course (as provided by the American Heart Association).

Successful defibrillation requires the provision of sufficient electrical current passage through the myocardium to interrupt the dysrhythmia, but not so much current as to cause morphologic damage.[7] The shocks should be given as soon as the defibrillator is available, both because the success rate decreases rapidly with time elapsed, and because electrical defibrillation is the treatment of choice in VF or pulseless VT.[7,11] With defibrillation, a substantial current of electrical energy is passed through the heart within a very short period of time. Grauer has emphasized the importance of lowering transthoracic resistance (TTR) to optimize the chance of conversion and minimize complications.[15] Many factors influence transthoracic resistance, including the chest-wall configuration, paddle pressure applied to the chest wall, the skin/paddle interface, paddle size and placement, the total number of and interval between shocks, and the phase of respiration. The practitioner can minimize TTR as follows.[10,11]

1 Use an electrode gel or disposable electrode pads.

2 Ensure correct paddle placement, i.e. the 'sternum' paddle below the clavicle and just to the right of the sternum and the 'apex' paddle lateral to the left nipple in the anterior axillary line.

3 Apply firm (approximately 25 lb) paddle pressure against the chest (in applying this pressure, think how much a 25-lb bag of sugar weighs).

4 Deliver the shock during exhalation (firm paddle pressure will aid forced exhalation).

TTR falls somewhat with successive shocks and with a shorter interval between shocks, so if the initial attempt is unsuccessful, minimizing the time to deliver the next shock is important.

The duration of ventricular fibrillation has a negative correlation with success rate.[11] The goal is speed when attempting defibrillation, since it is the single most important therapy that can be provided to the patient in VF or pulseless VT.[7,10,11] The underlying health of the myocardium and the environment in which it is found also influence success. Previously healthy hearts respond to defibrillation better than diseased ones. Hypoxia, acidosis, electrolyte imbalance, hypothermia and drug toxicity all render the fibrillating heart more resistant to therapy.[10,11]

With the introduction of automatic external defibrillators, basic life support (BLS)-trained hospital staff are encouraged to provide early electrical treatment for ventricular fibrillation (VF) and pulseless ventricular tachycardia (VT), even before the 'Code team' arrives with full advanced cardiac life support (ACLS) capabilities.[7-9,11] As distinct from manual monitor-defibrillators, which display the rhythm for the practitioner to interpret and act upon, these automated devices analyze the rhythm and advise 'shock' or 'no shock' depending upon the characteristics of the rhythm. It is up to the practitioner to determine unresponsiveness, lack of respiration and lack of pulse, and to apply the patches to the patient. The major advantage of this technology is the rapid availability of electrical therapy to the patient in VF or pulseless VT, thus providing a 'bridge' from cardiopulmonary resuscitation (CPR) to formal ACLS therapy. Non-physician BLS providers, in both prehospital and in-hospital settings, can readily be trained to operate this equipment, with a resulting improvement in survival rates.[11] This technology is ideal for freestanding imaging centers, and would also be appropriate for hospital-based imaging departments with ACLS Code-team backup.

Manual defibrillator operation is somewhat variable, depending on the machine, but some generalizations can be made. The power switches to the monitor and defibrillator sections may be separate or combined. If the patient is not already on an ECG monitor, most defibrillators provide a 'quick-look' feature that allows the paddles to act as ECG electrodes. The appropriate energy level is selected, and the capacitor is charged to that level. With the paddles correctly positioned as described above, the usual technique requires the practitioner to depress the firing buttons simultaneously on both paddles. Most monitor-defibrillators label the controls for simplicity of operation (e.g. 1, 2, 3), but the practitioner is advised to become familiar with the operation of the particular machine(s) that he or she may be called upon to use. Routine testing and documentation of the defibrillator at full output into a 50-ohm test load is recommended. In general, the procedure for manual defibrillation is as follows.[10,11]

1 Continue CPR *only until the defibrillator is ready*, i.e. do not delay defibrillation because of the need to perform CPR. CPR will need to be discontinued in order to confirm the rhythm without artifact from chest compressions.

2 Confirm that the rhythm is VF or pulseless VT, either selecting standard ECG leads or selecting the paddles as input electrodes. Possible pitfalls include motion artifact simulating VF, a lead off the patient, operator motion when using the paddles as leads, and selecting paddles or 'quick look' when the standard limb leads are attached to the patient.

3 Apply conductive gel or disposable pads, confirm that the defibrillator power is switched on, select the appropriate energy level, and charge the defibrillator.

4 Place the paddles as described above, with a slight 'twist' to distribute the conductive gel. Confirm that the rhythm is VF, and that all personnel are standing clear of the patient and anything that he or she is touching.

5 Apply firm paddle pressure and depress both buttons simultaneously.

6 Check the rhythm after each shock. Check for a pulse if there is a potentially perfusing rhythm on the monitor.

Synchronized cardioversion

The principle underlying synchronized cardioversion is to avoid delivering a shock during the 'vulnerable period', a period of approximately 30 ms in duration just before the apex of the T wave, during which the heart is most susceptible to electrically induced ventricular fibrillation.[10,11] This is distinct from defibrillation, which is timed only by the practitioner, and is therefore applied randomly with respect to the cardiac cycle. Synchronized cardioversion (sometimes called cardioversion) is performed by monitoring the patient with the ECG lead that shows a tall, upright R wave, which is sensed by the defibrillator when the appropriate controls are set. The machine then waits until it senses an R wave, and times the delivery of the shock so as to avoid the vulnerable period. It is most effective against dysrhythmias of re-entry origin, such as atrial flutter/fibrillation, PSVT and ventricular tachycardia. In general the procedure is as follows.[10,11]

1 Monitor the lead showing a tall, upright R wave. (In VT with rates over 200 beats/min and wide, bizarre QRS complexes, it may not be possible for the practitioner or the machine to discriminate between the R and T waves. In this case, proceed with unsynchronized defibrillation.

2 Activate the 'synch' switch and confirm that the machine is sensing the R waves. Charge the defibrillator to the desired energy level.

3 Apply gel or disposable pads, place the paddles, and ensure that all personnel are standing well clear.

4 Press and hold the buttons on each paddle. Unlike defibrillation, the machine will not deliver the stored energy to the paddles until the R wave is sensed.

5 Check the rhythm after each shock.

Autonomic nervous system physiology

A complete discussion of the autonomic nervous system is well beyond the intent or scope of this chapter, but a brief review is appropriate before consideration of emergency medications.[10,11] The sympathetic nervous system (SNS) and parasympathetic nervous system (PNS) comprise the autonomic nervous system, which is responsible for regulation of unconscious functions such as control of heart rate and blood pressure, intestinal motility, bladder control, and some hormonal activity (notably epinephrine release from the adrenal gland). Fibers of the preganglionic fibers of both the SNS and the PNS and the postganglionic fibers of the PNS mediate impulse formation by the release of acetylcholine, and are thus termed cholinergic. Postganglionic fibers of the SNS are mediated by norepinephrine release, and are termed adrenergic.

A balance between PNS and SNS tone generally exists, and promotes homeostasis at rest. Generalized stimulation of the SNS results in the classic 'fright or flight' response of tachycardia, raised blood pressure, pupilary dilatation, bronchial dilatation, anal sphincter contraction and inhibition of intestinal peristalsis. This is achieved through a combination of direct adrenergic innervation of target organs and epinephrine release from the adrenal gland. As a rule, stimulation of the PNS has the opposite effect, sometimes termed 'repose and repair'. Thus cholinergic stimulation results in slowing of the heart rate, a fall in blood pressure and resumption of peristalsis.

The heart, like many other organs, is innervated by both PNS and SNS fibers whose end-point effects are mediated by acetylcholine and norepinephrine, respectively.[10,11] The vagus nerve constitutes the direct PNS innervation of the heart, exerting its influence primarily on the SA node (slowed rate of spontaneous depolarization), and the AV node (prolonged AV conduction time). SNS innervation of the heart is mediated by adrenergic receptors located on cell surfaces, further divided into alpha-1, alpha-2, beta-1, and beta-2 receptors.

Alpha-1-adrenergic receptors are postsynaptic, located predominantly on the cellular surfaces of vascular smooth muscle. When stimulated, they produce vasoconstriction. Alpha-2 receptors, located on the presynaptic ends of the sympathetic neuron, inhibit further norepinephrine release when they are stimulated, thus functioning as an inhibitory feedback mechanism. For the purposes of the following discussion, 'alpha'-adrenergic stimulation will refer to alpha-1 receptors. Beta-1 adrenergic receptors are primarily located in the myocardium, and when stimulated cause an increase in the rate and strength of cardiac contractions (positive chronotropic and inotropic effects). Beta-2 receptors are found on vascular smooth muscle, where stimulation results in vasodilatation, and on bronchial smooth muscle, where stimulation causes bronchodilatation. Homeostasis of cardiac function and blood pressure control depends on a balance between PNS and SNS stimulation. Excess PNS or SNS tone can 'swing the pendulum' in one direction or the other, as can exogenous adrenergic agents (Tables 6.1 and 6.2).

Emergency medications

This section will present some basic pharmacology relating to medications commonly used in the treatment of contrast-related cardiac emergencies. Texts by Grauer,[10] Opie,[12] Kofke,[13] and Govani[14] are recommended for further reading. Unless otherwise specified, the doses stated are for adults.

Table 6.1   Adrenergic receptors – response of effector organs

Effector organ	Receptor type	Response
Heart	Beta	SA rate increased, AV conduction increased, contractility increased
Coronary arteries	Beta>alpha	Dilation>constriction
Peripheral arteries and veins	Alpha>beta	Constriction>dilation

Table 6.2   Adrenergic receptors – designation and effects

Designation	Location	Effect
Alpha 1	Vascular smooth muscle	Vasoconstriction
Alpha 2	Sympathetic neurons	Inhibits further norepinephrine release
Beta 1	Myocardium	Increased heart rate, contraction
Beta 2	Vascular smooth muscle Bronchial smooth muscle	Vasodilation Bronchodilation

Adenosine

Actions/indications   Adenosine is a naturally occurring substance that binds to cardiac receptors in the SA and AV nodes and results in decreased heart rate, depressed conduction, and increased refractoriness of the AV node. Its primary application is in the reliable and rapid termination of PSVT. It is very effective against re-entry atrial and nodal dysrhythmias and AV reciprocating tachycardias, but is not effective against atrial fibrillation or flutter, other than transiently to slow the ventricular response due to AV block. It may play a role in assisting diagnosis of some wide complex tachycardias by transiently increasing the degree of AV block, thereby unmasking underlying atrial activity.[15,18] It has an extremely short serum half-life of less than 5 s,[7] which may allow the dysrhythmia to recur, but also minimizes the duration of adverse effects.[6,7]

Adverse effects   Dyspnea (adenosine is a bronchoconstrictor), flushing, headache and occasional angina have been reported, but because the half-life is so short, these effects are transient, lasting less than 30–60 s.[12] Up to 50 per cent of patients will have transient, usually asymptomatic, dysrhythmias (PVCs, nonsustained VT, sinus pauses and AV block) immediately following SVT termination.[13]

Contraindications   Asthma, sick sinus syndrome, second- or third-degree AV block.

Dose Initial dose: 6-mg IV bolus (1–3 s). The effect on the AV node is rapid. If unsuccessful within 1–2 min, the repeat dose is 12 mg. If still unsuccessful, the 12-mg dose may be repeated after another 1–2 min, but if there is still no response, it is unlikely that the drug will be effective.[15]

Albuterol

Actions/indications Albuterol is a synthetic beta-2 selective agonist (with some beta-1 activity).[12] Its primary application in radiologic emergencies is for reversal of contrast-induced bronchospasm. It can be administered by metered-dose inhaler, thus delivering medication directly to the target organ (beta-2 receptors on bronchial smooth muscle).

Adverse effects With excessive dosages, tachycardia may occur because of the beta-1 component, but this is less of a problem than with aerosolized racemic epinephrine.

Contraindications Hypertension, tachycardia.

Dose One or two inhalations, repeated once in 1–2 min if needed. A maximum of four inhalations is suggested. Observe the patient for increased heart rate.

Atropine

Actions/indications Atropine sulfate is a parasympathetic blocking agent. Its primary application is in the acceleration of symptomatic sinus bradycardia, with additional uses in second- or third-degree AV block, slow idioventricular rhythm, and occasionally in asystole. It should not be given in asymptomatic bradycardia because of the potential risk of unmasking excessive underlying sympathetic tone.[10,11]

Adverse effects Pupilary dilatation, dry mouth, relatively unopposed sympathetic tone. The last item may be of importance in acute myocardial infarction or myocardial ischemia, where tachycardia may increase myocardial oxygen demand beyond the capacity of the coronary circulation.

Contraindications Normal sinus rhythm or tachycardia. Use with caution in acute myocardial infarction, due to the possibility of worsened ischemia with faster heart rate.[7]

Dose The recommended dose for hemodynamically unstable bradycardia is 1.0 mg IV every 3–5 min until the desired effect has been achieved, or a maximum dose of 0.04 mg/kg.[7] This may not be practicable in the severely symptomatic patient, in whom more frequent or higher doses are required because of the urgent need to re-establish adequate tissue perfusion. Atropine can also be given via endotracheal (ET) tube (as can epinephrine and lidocaine), but the pharmacokinetics are not as favorable as with IV administration. If given by ET tube, it should be administered in 1-mg increments.[10,11]

Dopamine

Actions/indications   Dopamine is a catecholamine-like agent with varying effects that are dependent on dose rate. At low infusion rates (1–2 μg/kg/min), so-called 'dopaminergic' effects predominate, characterized by dilatation of renal and mesenteric vascular beds, but there is little effect on heart rate or blood pressure.[10–14] At moderate (2–10 μg/kg/min) infusion rates, beta-adrenergic effects are observed, resulting in increased cardiac output without much elevation of blood pressure. At the same time, renal blood flow is relatively preserved, up to about 7.5 μg/kg/min. At high infusion rates above 10 μg/kg/min, alpha-adrenergic effects predominate and the drug behaves very much like epinephrine in this dose range. Thus the benefit of preserved renal/mesenteric blood flow is lost, and peripheral vasoconstriction, raised blood pressure and risk of tachyarrhythmias occur. Dopamine is used in cardiogenic and septic shock, bradycardia that is unresponsive to atropine, and electromechanical dissociation (EMD) (one form of pulseless electrical activity).

Adverse effects   As mentioned above, undesired elevation of blood pressure, PVCs and various tachyarrhythmias may occur. If the drug is infused through a peripheral vein and extravasated, local tissue ischemia or necrosis may ensue, so whenever possible administration through a central line is advised.

Contraindications   Ventricular arrhythmias and pheochromocytoma. Monamine oxidase (MAO) enzymatically inactivates norepinephrine, dopamine and serotonin. MAO inhibitors increase the concentration of catecholamines in the neuron and around the receptor, so the dopamine dose should be reduced to 10 per cent of what would normally be used.[12,13]

Dose   Mix one ampoule (200 mg) in 250 mL of D_5W and begin IV infusion at 1 μg/kg/min. Titrate to the desired clinical endpoint. Doses in the range 2–10 μg/kg/min generally have a beta-adrenergic effect, while at doses higher than 10 μg/min, alpha-adrenergic effects predominate.[7]

Epinephrine

Actions/Indications   Epinephrine is a potent, endogenously occurring catecholamine with both alpha- and beta-adrenergic effects.[10–13] At low concentrations, as may be seen with subcutaneous or slow IV infusion (1–2 μg/min), beta-adrenergic effects predominate, while at higher rates (2–10 μg/min) and bolus doses used in cardiac resuscitation, alpha-adrenergic effects predominate.[24] The alpha-adrenergic effects are highly desirable in the treatment of the arrested heart, because peripheral vasoconstriction raises blood pressure and favors blood supply to the coronary and cerebral circulations.[15,23] Coronary blood flow is facilitated by the rise in aortic diastolic pressure which occurs with peripheral vasoconstriction. Cerebral circulation is favored because the external carotid (a peripheral branch) is selectively vasoconstricted, forcing more blood into the internal carotid artery. The beta-adrenergic component results in a dramatic positive inotropic and chronotropic cardiac response. Because of shortened repolarization time and increased conduction velocities, epinephrine may theoretically facilitate defibrillation of VF. This may be evident as conversion of low-amplitude 'fine' VF to higher-amplitude 'coarse' VF, which appears to be more susceptible to defibrillation.[10,11] It is used in EMD in an attempt to increase myocardial contractility and blood pressure.[25–27] In asystole, epinephrine may be able to generate some electrical and mechanical activity.[10,11] Epinephrine is of great value in CPR due to preferential internal carotid perfusion.

Adverse effects   Epinephrine is a potent adrenergic agent and should be treated with due respect, especially in patients with established perfusing rhythms, in whom it will increase heart rate and blood pressure. Excessive administration may result in severe hypertension, ventricular tachyarrhythmias, increased myocardial oxygen demand, angina or left ventricular decompensation. Decreased renal blood flow may exacerbate renal injury in patients with pre-existing renal insufficiency. If epinephrine is extravasated outside a peripheral vein, local skin necrosis may occur.

Contraindications   Ventricular tachycardia, multiple PVCs, hypertension.[10–13] Use with caution in normotensive patients (e.g. in the treatment of some cases of anaphylaxis) and in patients on tricyclic antidepressants and MAO inhibitors.

Dose   For anaphylaxis give 1 mL (0.1 mg) of 1:10 000 solution over 2–5 min (e.g. 20 μg/min),[24] or 0.1–0.3 mg IV bolus if a larger dose is needed. (Note that adverse effects become more evident with larger, rapidly injected doses.)
   For cardiac resuscitation:

- IV bolus – 1.0 mg (10 mL of the 1:10 000 dilution) every 3–5 min as needed;[7]

- IV infusion – mix 1 mg in 250 mL D_5W, and begin infusion at 1 μg/min;

- endotracheal tube – 1.0–2.0 mg in 10 mL saline down the ET tube, followed by several (i.e. 5–10) forceful insufflations.[10,11]

Isoproterenol

Actions/indications   Isoproterenol is a synthetic catecholamine with beta-1 and beta-2 adrenergic effects. It is the most potent beta agonist available per microgram. At lower doses its beta-1 properties predominate, providing predominantly chronotropic effects. When higher doses are used its beta-2 effects become more predominant, and both positive cardiac inotropic effects and peripheral vasodilatation are observed. This may result in significantly increased cardiac output and demands on myocardial oxygen consumption. It is also a bronchodilator (beta-2 component). Therefore it may be of value in achieving a beta-adrenergic effect in patients on beta-blockers by 'overriding' the beta-blockade. It should be used, if at all, with extreme caution in patients with symptomatic bradycardia.[7]

Adverse effects   Myocardial ischemia (especially with coronary artery disease) secondary to increased cardiac output and possible hypotension from peripheral vasodilatation. Sinus or ventricular tachyarrhythmias are also observed.

Contraindications   Tachycardia, existing ventricular arrhythmia, angina. It should not be used in asystole, EMD or VF.[10]

Dose   Mix 1 mg in 250 mL D_5W and start infusion at 0.5 μg/min. The usual adult range is 0.5–20 μg/min.

Lidocaine

Actions/indications   Lidocaine is a local anesthetic agent with very useful antidysrhythmic properties that are largely confined to the ventricles, with very little antidysrhythmic effect on the atria or AV node.[7,10-14] It is the anti-arrhythmic drug of choice in ventricular ectopy, VT and VF.[7] However, in toxic doses it may depress automaticity of the sinus node. It preferentially decreases automaticity in ischemic ventricular tissue,[20] and is effective against orderly re-entrant dysrhythmias such as VT and bigeminy by improving conduction time. For lidocaine to be optimally effective, hypokalemia must be corrected. Since lidocaine is cleared by the liver, conditions that impair hepatic blood flow or function raise lidocaine blood levels and consequently the risk of toxicity. Such conditions include hepatitis, congestive heart failure (pulmonary edema), shock, advanced age and cimetidine use.[10] In these patients, dosages should be reduced to approximately half the usual dose. Indications for lidocaine in acute situations include suppression of frequent (more than 6–8/min), multifocal or ischemia-related PVCs, ventricular tachycardia and ventricular fibrillation.[10,11,13] For VF that recurs after initially successful defibrillation, lidocaine may be given before additional defibrillation attempts, but other causes of recurrent or refractory VF, such as hypoxia and acidosis, should be sought and corrected.

Adverse effects   Adverse effects are uncommon at therapeutic levels, toxicity usually occurring when therapeutic levels are exceeded. Inhibition of the sinus node with subsequent bradycardia and hypotension can occur, but the most common adverse reactions relate to the central nervous system. In approximate order of increasing blood level, these adverse effects include numbness, dizziness, drowsiness, dysarthria, confusion, seizures and respiratory arrest.[10]

Contraindications   Bradycardia may be exacerbated and escape beats (if present as a 'backup' mechanism) may be suppressed. Idioventricular rhythm may be converted to asystole, so lidocaine should never be given in third-degree AV block. Doses should be reduced in patients with suspected decreased hepatic function.

Dose   For PVC control and hemodynamically stable VT: loading dose is 1 mg/kg, repeated after 20 min if necessary. Maintenance dose is 1–4 mg/min, titrated to effect.

Nonperfusing VT and VF: Bolus of 1.5 mg/kg, with additional boluses of 0.5–1.5 mg/kg to a total of 3 mg/kg.[7] Infusion at 1–4 mg/min once a perfusing rhythm has been established.

Other medications

The drugs discussed above are those most often used in the initial treatment of acute cardiovascular emergencies related to adverse reactions to contrast media. Other cardiac medications, such as bretylium, digoxin, procainamide, propranolol and verapamil, may be necessary and can be used as second- or third-line treatment. The reader is referred to texts such as those by Grauer,[10] and Opie,[12] and to more specifically cardiac-related sources.[7,11,13,14,18,28,29]

Resuscitation algorithms

The practitioner who desires or requires a complete knowledge of, and skills in, the management of cardiopulmonary emergencies is urged to complete the American Heart Association's Advanced Cardiac Life Support (ACLS) course. The aim of this section is to present a simplified approach to the initial recognition and management of cardiac events that occur in radiology departments, with the assumption that full hospital Code-team backup or very rapid community-based ACLS services are available. As with prehospital delivery of emergency medical services, the key to improved survival of in-hospital cardiopulmonary arrest and preservation of neurologic function lies in the 'chain of survival' concept, namely prompt recognition of apnea and lack of pulse, rapid activation of a system that provides immediate basic life support (BLS) with CPR and rapidly follows that with external defibrillation (if available), and finally ACLS techniques.[4-6,10,11] Radiology department staff are in an ideal position to provide primary recognition and early management of cardiopulmonary arrest, transitional care (including external defibrillation) before the Code team arrives, and institution of ACLS protocols.

This section will deal with four 'rhythms' that are uniformly fatal if left untreated, namely ventricular fibrillation (VF), pulseless ventricular tachycardia, pulseless electrical activity (PEA), and asystole. Of these, the initial management is identical in two (VF and pulseless VT) and nearly identical in the other two (PEA and asystole). This further simplifies the initial management decisions that the practitioner must make. In addition, bradycardia will be discussed, not because of its lethality but because it is such a common event in most departments. In the algorithms that are included in this section, only the first few steps of resuscitation will be presented. It is assumed that the typical scenario is an inpatient or outpatient radiology department with rapid access to a Code team and effective communications systems that can summon help at the same time as instituting these measures. For departments that lack this level of backup, complete ACLS certification, training and equipment are suggested.

Before discussing each algorithm, a brief review of a general approach to the patient in acute cardiac arrest is in order. In general, the sequence of events begins with the 'ABCs' namely *airway*, *breathing* and *circulation*. The patient is assessed for unresponsiveness, and assistance (including a Code team) is summoned. *The importance of establishing and maintaining an intact airway cannot be overestimated: without an adequate airway and effective ventilations, all subsequent efforts will be futile.* If not contraindicated, the head and neck are positioned to open the airway, and the adequacy of spontaneous respiratory efforts is assessed. If necessary, two quick ventilations are given, and the carotid artery is checked for a pulse. If equipment and trained personnel are available, external defibrillation protocols are activated. If required, CPR (preferably two-person) is instituted. Continued advanced life support measures are instituted as soon as qualified personnel and equipment are available.

Bradycardia algorithm (Fig. 6.14)

As a rule, bradycardias of multiple etiologies lend themselves to algorithm discussion because of the similarities of treatment between sinus bradycardia, slow ventricular response due to AV block, and slow idioventricular rhythm. The key question to ask in any case of bradycardia is whether or not there is hemodynamic compromise (systolic BP less than 90 mmHg, altered mental status, syncope, etc.). If no hemodynamic compromise is evident, observation and correction of the underlying cause (e.g. pain resulting in increased parasympathetic tone) is all that is necessary. However, if the ventricular rate is very slow (e.g. less than 30

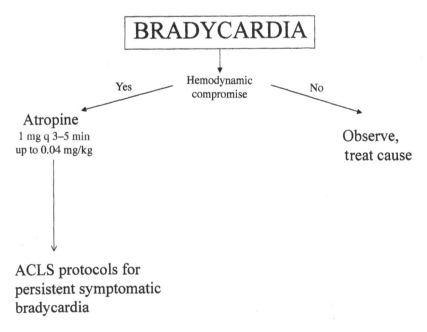

Figure 6.14 Bradycardia treatment algorithm.

beats/min), atropine should be considered because cardiac output is unlikely to remain sufficient for long, and ventricular escape beats may occur.

If there is hemodynamic compromise with bradycardia, a volume infusion of 500 mL normal saline or lactated Ringer's solution can be started (unless this is contraindicated by congestive heart failure (CHF) or pulmonary edema), and 1.0 mg of atropine IV can be given simultaneously, with repeated 0.5 to 1.0-mg increments up to a total of 2.0–3.0 mg,[10,11,24,30] or to 0.04 mg/kg.[7] As with any case of hemodynamic compromise, oxygen should be given to maximize tissue oxygenation. If there is concern about volume excess, the infusion should be decreased as soon as a satisfactory rate and pressure have been established. If the bradycardia is unresponsive to atropine, and the patient is still symptomatic, ACLS measures including chronotropic dopamine or epinephrine drips may be instituted and titrated to the desired ventricular rate.[7,10,13] As a last resort, a pacemaker may be required.[7,31–33]

Asystole algorithm (Fig. 6.15)

Asystole occurring in a procedural setting may in fact be profound bradycardia secondary to overwhelming parasympathetic tone,[10] as distinct from asystole occurring as a result of, for example, myocardial infarction. Obviously the former has a much better prognosis and, although it is tempting to use atropine first because of this, epinephrine is a better initial choice for asystole. Not only will epinephrine accelerate any sinus activity potentially present, but it is also the one drug that preferentially preserves cerebral and coronary blood flow during cardiac arrest and

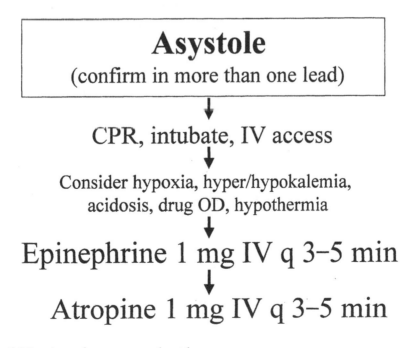

Figure 6.15   Asystole treatment algorithm.

CPR.[15,23] Since asystole is a fatal 'rhythm', giving high doses (1.0–1.5 mg) of epinephrine is a 'no-lose' approach.[34] Frequent use of epinephrine is advocated,[10,15] and it can be given IV or by ET every few minutes while CPR is in progress. As with any cardiopulmonary emergency, detailed attention to the airway and adequacy of ventilation/oxygenation are of paramount importance in order to provide adequate tissue oxygenation and to facilitate respiratory correction of metabolic acidosis, both of which will improve the environment of the myocardium and favor successful conversion. Bicarbonate administration should ideally be guided by arterial blood gas determination.

On occasion, 'fine' ventricular fibrillation may resemble a flat-line ECG if the machine gain setting is too low or the fibrillatory waves are perpendicular to the ECG lead that is being observed. Thus it is necessary to confirm asystole in at least two leads (if using quick-look paddles, rotate the paddle placement through 90 degrees) and to check that there is adequate gain on the monitor before concluding that there is no cardiac electrical activity. In addition, epinephrine may 'coarsen' fibrillatory waves to a sufficient magnitude that they become visible on the monitor,[10] and once they have been identified, defibrillation may commence.

Routine shocking of asystole is strongly discouraged because shocks have demonstrated no improvement in asystole and, in the uncommon event that the latter is the result of raised parasympathetic tone, the added parasympathetic discharge associated with electrical shock would only worsen the situation.[7]

The similarity of the asystole and PEA treatment algorithms is noteworthy. Intubation, IV access, CPR and epinephrine are the primary elements of management of both entities. In addition, a search for any identifiable underlying or contributing factors should be made, and these should be corrected if possible.

Pulseless electrical activity (PEA) algorithm (Fig. 6.16)

By definition this is a non-perfusing rhythm characterized by the absence of a pulse in the presence of organized cardiac electrical activity. The term includes primary electromechanical dissociation (EMD), which results from intrinsic failure of myocardial contractility and carries a poor prognosis despite vigorous therapy.[25–27] Secondary EMD results from profound alterations in the loading conditions of the myocardium, and if these can be identified and corrected in a timely manner, the prognosis is much better. As in asystole, epinephrine is the initial drug of choice because of its influence on the preservation of coronary and cerebral blood flow and its potent inotropic cardiac effect. The usual dose of epinephrine would be 1.0 mg IV (10 mL of the 1:10 000 dilution).[7,10,34]

There are a number of potentially reversible causes of PEA which should be searched for and treated if possible. These include inadequate ventilation/oxygenation, hypovolemia, septic shock, anaphylaxis (e.g. contrast reaction), pericardial tamponade, tension pneumothorax (PT), massive pulmonary embolus (PE), severe metabolic or respiratory acidosis, and electrolyte imbalance (e.g. hypokalemia).[7,10,11,25–27] (Hypothermia is an additional potentially reversible cause of PEA that will not be discussed here.) Even without an obvious cause, a bolus

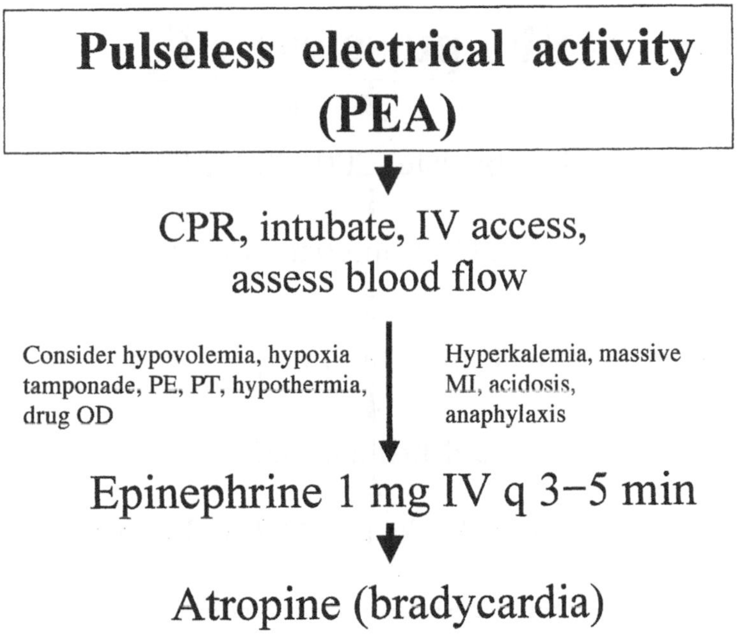

> ## Pulseless electrical activity (PEA)

↓

CPR, intubate, IV access,
assess blood flow

Consider hypovolemia, hypoxia
tamponade, PE, PT, hypothermia,
drug OD

Hyperkalemia, massive
MI, acidosis,
anaphylaxis

↓

Epinephrine 1 mg IV q 3–5 min

↓

Atropine (bradycardia)

Figure 6.16   Pulseless electrical activity (PEA) treatment algorithm.

infusion of 500 mL normal saline or lactated Ringer's solution has been recommended.[10] This may improve filling pressures in hypovolemic, septic, cardiogenic and anaphylactic shock and result in some improvement in cardiac output. For PEA that is unresponsive to bolus epinephrine and volume infusion, a dopamine drip or epinephrine drip may buy some additional time to search for and correct an underlying cause. Again, note the similarity to the asystole algorithm (Fig. 6.15).

Ventricular fibrillation/pulseless VT algorithm (VF/VT) (Fig. 6.17)

The single most effective treatment for the patient in VF or pulseless VT is early defibrillation. [4-6,10,11] The greatest impact on patient outcome can be expected when there is a coordinated effort by the practitioners closest to the patient (in this case, the radiology personnel) and those trained in automatic or manual defibrillation and ACLS techniques. To be optimally effective, the defibrillator and all associated oxygenation, ventilation and suction apparatus, as well as resuscitative medications, need to be immediately available. Although intubation, IV access and pharmacologic methods are all important, the initial focus should be on establishing the diagnosis of VF and rapid defibrillation. The first three shocks are delivered in a stacked sequence, one after the other, with no pause to administer medications, search for pulse or perform CPR.[7] The practitioners should evaluate the rhythm for persistent VF/VT after each shock (during recharging), and only remove the paddles and check for a pulse if there is a non-VF/VT rhythm on the monitor.[7] If VF/VT persists after the first stacked series of three shocks, then CPR is instituted, the patient is intubated and, if not already available, IV access is established.

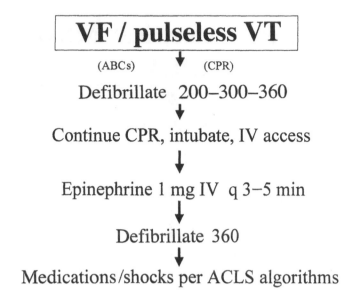

Figure 6.17 Ventricular fibrillation/pulseless ventricular tachycardia treatment algorithm.

Early application of electrical energy in VF or pulseless VT is the single most important action the practitioner can take for the patient. Defibrillation is the only effective treatment available, the chances of success decrease with time, and VF tends to deteriorate to asystole within a few minutes.[7] The rationale of starting defibrillation at a modest energy level and progressing upward is that somewhat fewer complications (e.g. asystole, heart block) may occur at the lower energy levels, and it is possible that the rhythm may convert at a lower energy level.[10,15] If this is unsuccessful, subsequent shocks at higher energy levels and at close intervals maximize the current delivered to the heart, presumably due in part to lowered transthoracic resistance in response to subsequent shocks.[10,11] As with asystole and EMD, frequent use of epinephrine is advocated because of its beneficial effects of preservation of coronary and cerebral blood flow, and positive inotropic and chronotropic cardiac effects.[15] One should allow sufficient time for the epinephrine to reach the central circulation while CPR is in progress before subsequent defibrillation attempts are made. It should be remembered that epinephrine and lidocaine may be given by endotracheal (ET) tube if IV access cannot be established. For endotracheal administration, if the initial dose of 1 mg is not effective, the dose is increased to 2 to 3 times the usual IV dose, e.g. 2–3 mg.[10] Additional epinephrine may be given after other medications if necessary. Likewise, there is no limit on the number of times that defibrillation may be attempted.[10]

If the patient is refractory to epinephrine and defibrillations, the team is dealing with refractory or persistent VF. Further resuscitative measures as specified in the ACLS protocols should be instituted. As was discussed in the introduction to this section, it is assumed that radiology practices associated with hospitals will have immediate access to Code teams.

Summary

As radiologists take on a larger role in the management of complex clinical problems, there is a need for increased responsibility in the prevention and management of iatrogenic or spontaneously occurring emergencies. As the complexity and risk of radiologic procedures increase, practitioners will need to hone skills to prevent, identify and treat these complications. Preprocedural evaluation, patient preparation, intraprocedural care, monitoring, airway management and dysrhythmia recognition/management are important aspects of caring for patients in radiology environments.

References

1. Society of Cardiovascular and Interventional Radiology. *Standards of Practice*. Fairfax, VA: Society of Cardiovascular and Interventional Radiology.

2. Capek P, McLean GK, Berkowitz HD. Femoropopliteal angioplasty: factors influencing long-term success. *Circulation* 1991; **83** (Suppl. I): 70–80.

3. Hertzer NR. The natural history of peripheral vascular disease: implications for its management. *Circulation* 1991; **83** (Suppl. I): 12–19.

4. Montgomery WH. Prehospital cardiac arrest: the chain of survival concept. *Annals of the Academy of Medicine, Singapore* 1992; **21**: 69–72.

5. Cummins RO, Ornato JP, Thies WH *et al.* Improving survival from sudden cardiac arrest: the 'chain of survival' concept. *Circulation* 1991; **83**: 1832–47.

6. Hunt RC, McCabe JB, Hamilton GC, Krohmer JR. Influence of emergency medical services systems and prehospital defibrillation on survival of sudden cardiac death victims. *American Journal of Emergency Medicine* 1989; **7**: 68–82.

7. Emergency Cardiac Care Committee and Subcommittees of the American Heart Association. Guidelines for cardiopulmonary resuscitation and emergency cardiac care. I. Introduction. *Journal of the American Medical Association* 1992; **268**: 2172–83.

8. Shuster M, Keller JL. Effect of fire department first-responder automated defibrillation. *Annals of Emergency Medicine* 1993; **22**: 721–7.

9. Schrading WA, Stein S, Eitel DR *et al.* An evaluation of automated defibrillation and manual defibrillation by emergency medical technicians in a rural setting. *American Journal of Emergency Medicine* 1993; **11**: 125–30.

10. Grauer K, Cavallaro D. ACLS, *Certification preparation and a comprehensive review, 2nd edn.* St Louis, MO: C.V. Mosby Co., 1987.

11. Cummins R, ed. *Textbook of advanced cardiac life support*. Dallas, TX: American Heart Association, 1994.

12. Opie LH. *Drugs for the heart*. Philadelphia, PA: W.B. Saunders & Co., 1991.

13. Kofke WA, Levy JH, eds. *Postoperative critical care procedures of the Massachusetts General Hospital*. New York: Little, Brown and Co., 1986.

14. Govoni LE, Hayes JE. *Drugs and nursing implications*. New York: Appleton and Lange, 1988.

15. Grauer K, Cavalloro D, Gums J. New developments in cardiopulmonary resuscitation. *American Family Physician* 1991; **43**: 832–44.

16. Trunkey D, ed. *Advanced trauma life support*. Chicago, IL: American College of Surgeons, Committee on Trauma, 1984.

17. Caruso AC. Supraventricular tachycardia: changes in management. *Postgraduate Medicine* 1991; **90**: 73–6, 79–82.

18. Sager PT, Bhandari AK. Narrow complex tachycardias, differential diagnosis and management. *Cardiology Clinics* 1991: **9**: 619–40.

19. Arai A, Kron J. Current management of the Wolff-Parkinson-White syndrome. *Western Journal of Medicine* 1990: **152**: 383–91.

20. Wesle RC, Resh W, Zimmerman D. Reconsiderations of the routine and preferential use of lidocaine in the emergent treatment of ventricular arrhythmias. *Critical Care Medicine* 1991; **19**: 1439–44.

21. Zaim S, Walter PF. Diagnosis and treatment of ventricular tachycardia. *Heart Disease and Stroke* 1992; **1**: 141–7.

22. Chakko S, de Marchena E, Kessler KM, Myerburg RJ. Ventricular arrhythmias in congestive heart failure. *Clinical Cardiology* 1989; **12**: 525–30.

23. Waller DG, Robertson CE. Role of sympathomimetic amines during cardiopulmonary resuscitation. *Resuscitation* 1991; **22**: 181–90.

24. Bush WH, Swanson DP. Acute reactions to intravascular contrast media: types, risk factors, recognition and specific treatement. *American Journal of Roentgenology* 1991; **157**: 1153–61.

25. Kothari SS. Electromechanical dissociation: treatable causes of a dire cardiac emergency. *Postgraduate Medicine* 1991; **90**: 75–8.

26. Cripps T, Camm J. The management of electromechanical dissociation. *Resuscitation* 1991; **22**: 173–80.

27. Charlap S, Kahlam S, Lichstein E, Frishman W. Electromechanical dissociation: diagnosis, physiology, management. *American Heart Journal* 1989; **118**: 355–60.

28. Haft JI, Habbab MA. Treatment of atrial arrhythmias: effectiveness of verapamil when preceded by calcium infusion. *Archives of Internal Medicine* 1986; **146**: 1085–7.

29. Salerno DM, Dias VC, Kleiger RE, *et al.* Intravenous verapamil for treatment of multifocal atrial tachycardia with and without calcium pretreatment. *Annals of Internal Medicine* 1987; **107**: 623–5.

30. Bush WH, McClennan BL, Swanson DP. Contrast media reactions: prediction, prevention and treatment. *Postgraduate Radiology* 1993; **13**: 137–47.

31. Wood M, Ellenbogen KA. Bradyarrhythmias, emergency pacing, and implantable defibrillation devices. *Critical Care Clinics* 1989; **5**: 551–68.

32. Kirschenbaum LP, Eisenkraft JB, Mitchell J, Hillel Z. Transthoracic pacing for the treatment of severe bradycardia during induction of anesthesia. *Journal of Cardiothoracic Anesthesia* 1989; **3**: 329–32.

33. Fitzpatrick A, Sutton R. A guide to temporary pacing. *British Medical Journal* 1992; **304**: 365–9.

34. Ornato JP. High-dose epinephrine during resuscitation. A word of caution (editorial). *Journal of the American Medical Association* 1991; **265**: 1160–61.

7 Sedation, analgesia and patient observation in interventional radiology

Jeffrey P. Quam and Michael A. Bettmann

Over the past few years, the scope of practice of diagnostic radiology has broadened dramatically. Coinciding with this increased capacity to image has been an increase in the ability of the radiologist to perform image-guided interventional procedures for both diagnostic and therapeutic purposes. These developments have had a tremendous positive impact on the practice of modern medicine. As a consequence of this trend, radiologists now have greater responsibility in the management of interventional patients. In addition to successfully performing the procedure itself, radiologists must prevent or limit the physical and emotional suffering of their patients. The utilization of various pharmacologic agents can achieve this by relieving anxiety, providing sedation and alleviating pain. The development of new, short-acting and reliable drugs has made sedation and analgesia simpler and safer. Consequently, the responsibility of managing these patients has been passed from anesthesiologists to radiologists. In using these agents the radiologist must be prepared to recognize and address the risks involved in their use. Although the radiologist is primarily responsible, well-trained and experienced radiology nurses and technologists must be engaged in all aspects of the procedure.

The American Society of Anesthesiologists has defined several levels of depressed consciousness,[1] as listed in Table 7.1. This chapter will focus on the administration of 'conscious sedation', given the premise that situations requiring 'deep sedation' or 'general anesthesia' will have an anesthetist or anesthesiologist in attendance. Nevertheless, it must be recognized that an attempt to induce conscious sedation can lead to unexpected deep sedation or even general anesthesia.

Many tasks must be addressed in the successful performance of sedation-assisted interventional procedures. Prior to the procedure, a clinical evaluation of the

Table 7.1   American Association of Anesthesiologists' levels of depressed consciousness[1]

Conscious sedation:	A minimally depressed level of consciousness that retains the patient's ability to maintain a patent airway independently and continuously, and to respond appropriately to physical stimulation and verbal commands.
Deep sedation:	A controlled state of depressed consciousness or unconsciousness from which the patient is not easily aroused and is unable to respond purposefully to physical stimulation or verbal commands. This may be accompanied by loss of protective reflexes and an inability to maintain a patent airway independently.
General anesthesia:	A controlled state of unconsciousness accompanied by a loss of protective reflexes, including loss of the ability to maintain a patent airway independently or to respond purposefully to physical stimulation or verbal commands.

prospective patient must be performed. During the procedure, appropriate pharmacologic administration and patient monitoring is necessary. Following the procedure, close patient care and continued monitoring are needed to ensure safe recovery of the patient. None of these three phases of patient care can be addressed properly without a thorough understanding of the various pharmacologic agents that are available for sedation and analgesia.

Pharmacology

The goals of preprocedural and procedural pharmacologic management for patients undergoing percutaneous interventional procedures are listed in Table 7.2. Intravenous administration is most appropriate for radiologic procedures, even though many of the agents can be administered using other routes (e.g. oral, rectal or intramuscular). When given intravenously, the agents have a more specific, predictable onset of action, and their effects are more easily and accurately titratable. Inhalational anesthetics are beyond the scope of this text, and should only be administered by professionals with specific training in anesthesia. The drugs used to treat anaphylactoid reactions to contrast material are addressed in Chapters 3, 4 and 6 of this book.

Ideally, the sedative and analgesic agents administered by radiologists during interventional procedures should have the following characteristics: they should act rapidly (to allow predictability of their onset of action), have a short effective biological half-life (thus affording easy titratability to the desired clinical effect), and be quickly eliminated (ensuring a timely, safe recovery for the patient). These qualities give the agents a good safety profile, allowing maximal therapeutic effect and minimal toxicity. The goals of conscious sedation, various drug classes and the clinical effects of these classes are outlined in Table 7.2.

Table 7.2 Goals of preprocedural and procedural pharmacologic management for patients undergoing percutaneous interventional procedures

Clinical goal	Drug class
Relief of anxiety	Benzodiazepines
Sedation	Benzodiazepines, narcotics, antihistamines
Amnesia	Benzodiazepines
Local analgesia	Aromatic amines (lidocaine, bupivacaine)
Systemic analgesia	Narcotics
Decreased secretions	Antihistamines, anticholinergics

Numerous agents can be used for the general goal of conscious sedation, and a comprehensive discussion of all of them is beyond the scope of this chapter. The following section will discuss several commonly used agents based on their desired clinical effects, and is therefore divided into subsections on sedatives, local anesthetics, systemic anesthetics and reversal agents. As can be seen in Table 7.2, some drug classes may have more than one desired effect, and these agents will therefore be discussed in more than one subsection.

Each subsection includes a brief history of the prototypical agent and the mechanism of action of the drug class. This is followed by a discussion of several specific agents in each class that offer advantages relative to the prototypical agent or other agents within the class. Some readers may disagree with regard to the specific agents selected here. This is both expected and appropriate, as the list of agents discussed is not meant to be exhaustive. Regardless of the pharmacologic armamentarium that is ultimately selected, it is essential that the radiologist be familiar with his or her favored drugs and the treatment of their side-effects.

Sedatives

The current use of intravenous sedation (Table 7.3) evolved as a modification of the induction of general anesthesia using barbiturates and opiates. However, barbiturates have suboptimal pharmacokinetics with a prolonged half-life (e.g. amobarbital and phenobarbital have elimination half-lives of up to 40 h and 120 h, respectively). They also cause significant, dose-related cardiovascular and CNS depression.[2] Another drawback of barbiturates is their potential to decrease the pain threshold at lower, sedative doses. The popularity of intravenous sedation techniques increased rapidly with the development and introduction of the benzodiazepines in the mid-1960s. Of the synthetic benzodiazepines that were evaluated for their efficacy as skeletal muscle relaxants in 1957, chlordiazepoxide was the first found to have sedative-hypnotic effects as well.[3] Subsequently, diazepam (Valium®) was approved for use in 1961, lorazepam (Ativan®) in 1971 and midazolam (Versed®) in 1976.

The primary mode of action of the benzodiazepines is through facilitation of the gamma-aminobutyric acid (GABA) system in the CNS. This system is the largest and most powerful inhibitory system in the brain. Benzodiazepine-binding sites are

Table 7.3 Sedative agents

Drug	Initial dose	Maximum dose	Onset of action	Duration of action
Diazepam	2–5 mg	0.2 mg/kg	3–5 min	1–2 h (second peak at 5–8 h)
Midazolam	0.5–1 mg	5 mg	2–3 min	30–60 min
Propofol	(see text)	(see text)	(see text)	(see text)
Diphenhydramine	25–50 mg	100 mg	5–8 min	2–4 h
Lorazepam	2–5 mg	0.1 mg/kg	3–5 min	6–8 h

The doses listed are suggested when the agent is given alone to a healthy patient. Doses must be modified when used in combination and in patients with relevant comorbidity.

For all of the agents discussed, the package insert should be consulted for a full description of the doses, pharmacokinetics and contraindications.

found throughout the CNS, but are most numerous in the cerebral cortex and least numerous in the spinal cord. Benzodiazepines do not act directly at GABA-receptor sites, but instead enhance the binding of GABA to its receptors.[4] This enhances the GABA-mediated conductance of chloride through the cell membrane.[5] Through direct GABA potentiation, benzodiazepines enhance the degree of general CNS inhibition.

Benzodiazepines replaced barbiturates as the sedative of choice mainly because of their remarkably low capacity to produce the fatal CNS depression seen with barbiturates.[6] In addition to their sedative properties, benzodiazepines also became popular as a result of their efficacy with regard to anxiolytic effects, combined with minimal general depression of the CNS.[7] Benzodiazepines were also shown to promote amnesia by preventing memory consolidation.[8] Thus, with this single drug class, three of the goals (anxiolysis, sedation and amnesia) listed in Table 7.2 are achieved. However, it must be emphasized that benzodiazepines provide very little, if any, analgesia.[9] If used alone, the patient will be sedated but will still experience pain during the procedure. Thus an analgesic should almost always be given in conjunction with a benzodiazepine.

In healthy patients, benzodiazepines have only slight respiratory depressive effects when used alone and appear primarily to block the ventilatory response to hypoxia.[10] However, the addition of a narcotic markedly increases the risk of hypoxemia.[11] Respiratory depression is mainly due to depression of both the hypoxic and the hypercapnic respiratory centers in the brainstem. General skeletal muscle relaxation may also contribute to the respiratory depression.[10] A recent study by Bailey et al. suggested that blunting of the ventilatory response to hypoxia occurred earlier and to a greater degree than did the response to hypercarbia, when a benzodiazepine and narcotic were given.[11] In theory, therefore, arterial oxygen partial pressure (PO_2) may drop to critically low levels before increased ventilation would be stimulated by a sufficiently high blood CO_2 tension.

Benzodiazepines can also cause mild systemic arterial hypotension, usually with an appropriate increase in heart rate. With diazepam and lorazepam, the drop in blood pressure is due to a mild negative inotropic effect.[12] Hypotension with midazolam is a consequence of decreased peripheral vascular resistance. Sensitivity to both respiratory and cardiovascular depressive effects is increased in elderly patients.[13]

Following its introduction, diazepam became the mainstay of intravenous sedation for many years. It is still commonly used today but is more often employed as an oral medication for long-term management of anxiety and seizure prevention. For intravenous sedation, diazepam has been superseded by midazolam for several practical reasons. Both diazepam and lorazepam are lipophilic and insoluble in water. This lipophilicity is desirable in that it allows a rapid effect on the CNS, but it requires that the drugs be combined with an organic solvent (e.g. ethyl alcohol, propylene glycol or sodium benzoate) before intravenous injection. These solvents cause local pain on injection and, more importantly, they can induce thrombophlebitis. Midazolam is chemically distinct, with an imidazole ring that is open, ionized and water-soluble when injected, and thus has neither of these disturbing side-effects. The ring then closes upon injection, at physiologic pH, and midazolam regains a lipophilicity that still allows a rapid effect on the CNS.

At equisedative doses, midazolam produces a greater amnestic effect and causes less respiratory depression than either diazepam or lorazepam.[14,15] Titration of midazolam to achieve the appropriate desired effect is more reliable. Midazolam is highly lipophilic, has the shortest effective half-life of any of the benzodiazepines, and has little significant prolonged or unpredictable effect from active metabolites or enterohepatic circulation. Diazepam has the disadvantage of greater variability in patient response to its sedative and anxiolytic properties, partly due to an extremely long-acting metabolite of diazepam (N-desmethyldiazepam). It also has a second plasma concentration peak that occurs 5–8 h after injection and is probably due to enterohepatic circulation.[16] Lorazepam is the least lipophilic benzodiazepine and therefore only penetrates the CNS slowly. This limited lipophilicity also results in a smaller volume of distribution and thus a prolonged effective duration.[17]

Propofol (Diprivan®) is a fairly new sedative-hypnotic agent that was introduced as an anesthesia-induction agent. It is formulated as an aqueous emulsion in soybean oil, and is given intravenously in bolus form and/or as a maintenance infusion. The usual initial dose of propofol is 100 μg/kg body weight, over 3 to 5 min. Effectiveness is then maintained with a constant infusion dose of 25–75 μg/kg/min. The need for constant maintenance infusion makes the use of propofol impractical for many radiology suites. Like other sedatives, it may cause respiratory depression and decreased cardiac output. Nevertheless, it has increased in popularity as a sedating agent for several reasons. It has a very rapid onset of action and an ultra-short half-life, giving fast emergence from sedation. It also has an anti-emetic effect.[18,19] Direct comparisons have shown a more rapid return to baseline with propofol than with midazolam.[20,21] A recent prospective study of conscious sedation during interventional neuroradiology procedures demonstrated the advantages of propofol, and also showed no subjective difference in patient satisfaction when using propofol in lieu of midazolam.[22] Like benzodiazepines, propofol does not have any analgesic properties, and thus should be used in combination with an analgesic during interventional procedures. The aqueous–oil emulsion does cause some local pain on injection, but there is no risk of thrombophlebitis as is seen with diazepam. This infusion pain can be treated either by local lidocaine infiltration or with systemic analgesics.[23] A final common, but harmless, side-effect of propofol is a temporary green discoloration of the patient's urine.

Antihistamines (specifically H_1-antagonists) are also useful as sedative agents, although they are generally less effective than benzodiazepines. All H_1-antagonists can bind to CNS receptors and cause varying levels of CNS depression, resulting in reduced alertness, slowed reaction times and somnolence.[24] The ethanolamines, a subclass which includes diphenhydramine (Benadryl®), are particularly effective in providing sedation. Antihistamines given systemically provide no analgesia, but do appear to potentiate the analgesic effects of narcotics. The greatest advantage of antihistamines is that, unlike benzodiazepines, there is no increased risk of respiratory or cardiovascular depression when they are used in combination with a narcotic. Thus they should be considered as the sedative of choice when being administered to patients with respiratory or cardiovascular compromise. Antihistamines have the added advantage of having anticholinergic effects,[24] which help to decrease oral and gastric secretions and reduce the risk of aspiration in patients who are undergoing procedures.

Local anesthetics

Local anesthetics should be the first-line choice of drug for pain relief during percutaneous interventional procedures. Insufficient local anesthesia should not be compensated for by higher doses of systemic analgesics. Although adequate doses of correctly administered local anesthetics may lead to systemic complications, the risk of toxicity is much greater when excess systemic analgesics are given.

The first agent to be used as a local anesthetic was the alkaloid cocaine, found in the leaves of the shrub *Erythroxlon coca*. Nieman was the first to isolate the pure alkaloid in 1860, at which time he noted its bitter taste and numbing effect on his tongue. In 1905, Einhorn *et al.* created the first synthetic cocaine analogue, procaine (Novacaine®), which became the prototype for local anesthetics.[25] Lidocaine (Xylocaine®) and bupivacaine (Marcaine®, Sensorcaine®), both of which are aromatic amines, are now the most commonly used local anesthetics.

Local anesthetics interfere with the sodium channels of the nerve-cell membrane. Under normal circumstances, a slight depolarization of the cell membrane generates a large transient increase in the permeability of the membrane to sodium. By blocking this rapid influx of sodium, local anesthetics increase the threshold of excitability and blunt the rate of increase in action potential. These factors thus decrease the probability of propagation of an action potential along the nerve fiber. The sodium channel must be active and open to allow the anesthetic to interfere with the channel's function. Although local anesthetics are non-specific nerve depressants (motor, sensory or autonomic), sensory nerve function is blocked earliest, because sensory neurons are the most rapidly firing type. Lidocaine was introduced in 1948 and is currently the most commonly used local anesthetic.[26] It replaced procaine partly as a result of the decreased incidence of anaphylactoid reactions associated with its use. Lidocaine also provides a more prolonged anesthesia than does procaine.

Large doses of lidocaine can cause CNS side-effects including dizziness, paresthesias, seizures and induction of coma.[27] The most lethal complications of excess doses are ventricular fibrillation and cardiac arrest.[28] These complications most often occur as a result of accidental intravenous administration, and care must be taken to avoid intravascular injection. Such complications can also occur as a result of very large doses of non-vascular lidocaine, but are very rare below the maximum dose of 5 mg/kg (0.5 mL/kg of 1 per cent solution). If the formulation includes a vasoconstricting agent (e.g. epinephrine), the local anesthetic action is both potentiated and prolonged. This is due to a decrease in the rate of systemic resorption of the agent from the site of injection, and this also decreases the frequency of systemic complications. However, epinephrine should not be added when infiltrating tissues that are supplied by end-arteries (e.g. fingers, toes, nose, ears or penis). Since these regions lack sufficient collateral arteries, ischemic necrosis may result from the vasoconstriction.

If the percutaneous procedure is anticipated to be prolonged, or if it results in placement of a temporary catheter in an area of tenderness, bupivacaine can be used as an alternative or adjunct to lidocaine. Bupivacaine is a longer-acting amide local anesthetic. However, this longer action comes at a price. In relatively low concentrations, bupivacaine slows cardiac conductivity and decreases contractility.[29] Lethal cardiovascular collapse is much more common with bupivacaine than with lidocaine.[30] Consequently, the maximum dose of bupivacane is only 2.5 mg/kg. Therefore, the maximum single dose for an average adult is about 70 mL of the 0.25 per cent solution, or 35 mL of the 0.5 per cent solution.

Both of these agents are acidic at physiologic pH, and consequently cause local pain upon tissue infiltration. Buffering with sodium bicarbonate minimizes this side-effect.[31] The mixing is done at a volumetric ratio of 10:1 (lidocaine: bicarbonate). If the formulation is stored mixed, the local anesthetic effect will decrease after approximately 1 week. Thus the mixing is optimally performed at the time of injection. It has also been shown that warming the lidocaine may decrease the painful sensation noted with injection.[32]

Antihistamines show varying levels of effectiveness as local anesthetics.[33] Infiltration of 1 per cent diphenhydramine appears to be as effective as a 1 per cent lidocaine solution. However, it has been reported that antihistamines cause greater local pain upon injection.[33] Nevertheless, in patients with a known allergy to lidocaine or severe cardiovascular disease, antihistamines serve as an effective alternative local anesthetic.

Systemic analgesics (Table 7.4)
In many cases, despite appropriate and complete local anesthesia, some patients may still suffer pain associated with the procedure. This occurs for a variety of reasons. Some cases (e.g. biliary stent placement, arterial angioplasty) require significant and prolonged manipulations involving several wires and catheters. Organ

Table 7.4 Systemic analgesics

Drug	Initial dose	Maximum dose	Onset of action	Duration of action
Morphine	3–5 mg	0.2 mg/kg	8–10 min	3–4 h
Meperidine	30–60 mg	2 mg/kg	5–8 min	2–3 h
Fentanyl	25–50 μg	3 μg/kg/h	1 min	30–60 min
Sufentanil	3–6 μg	Titrate slowly	< 1 min	15–30 min
Alfentanil	100–300 μg	Titrate slowly	< 1 min	20–40 min

The doses listed are suggested when the agent is given alone to a healthy patient. Doses must be modified when used in combination and in patients with relevant comorbidity.

For all of the agents discussed, the package insert should be consulted for a full description of the doses, pharmacokinetics and contraindications.

capsules and many specific surface membranes (e.g., pleura, periosteum) are difficult or impossible to anesthetize with local anesthetic infiltration. In these circumstances, the addition of systemic analgesics for patient comfort outweighs the risks of their use.

Just as the effects of benzodiazepines are limited to anxiolysis and amnesia, without analgesia, narcotics are most effective as analgesics but have little anxiolytic or amnestic effect. Thus the two agents are commonly used in combination. The word 'narcotic' is non-specific and, in its purest application, denotes any agent that produces stupor or sleepiness. Nevertheless, by convention the word usually refers to the opiates and opioids, as will be the case in this chapter. The terms 'opiate' and 'opioid' should not be used interchangeably. Opiates (e.g. morphine, codeine) are derived directly from raw opium or are semisynthetic morphine analogues, whereas opioids (e.g. meperidine, fentanyl) are totally synthetic drugs whose effects are similar to those of opiates. Both of these terms are derived from the Greek word 'opion', meaning 'juice', referring to the juice of the poppy, *Papaver somniferum*, from which opium is derived.[34]

The earliest documented account of the use of opium was in Sumeria, around 4600 BC. Its use quickly spread to Arabia, the Orient and Europe. In 1806, Friedrich Serteurner isolated the first of many distinct opium components. This gave him the right to name it, which he did after Morpheus, the Greek god of dreams. Morphine is thus considered to be the prototypical narcotic. The other two medically useful derivatives of opium are codeine, which was isolated in 1832, and the vasodilator papaverine, which was isolated in 1848. Subsequently, many semisynthetic and synthetic analogues have been developed.

Opiate/opioid receptors were described simultaneously by several separate investigators in 1973.[35-37] There are many classes and subclasses of receptors, and some knowledge of these is helpful in understanding the effects of various opioids. The most important classes in relation to analgesia are mu-receptors and kappa-receptors. Mu-1-receptors mostly lie in the brain, and their stimulation results in supraspinal analgesia and slight euphoria. Mu-2-receptors are found in the cerebral cortex, medial thalamus, periaqueductal gray matter and gastrointestinal (GI) tract. Stimulation of mu-2-receptors causes many of the negative side-effects, including respiratory depression, decreased GI motility, nausea and vomiting, and drug dependence. Kappa-1-receptors mediate analgesia at the spinal level and also induce some sedation. Kappa-3-receptors are the most numerous receptors in the brain, and participate in supraspinal analgesia.

The analgesic effects of these narcotics are due to agonist action at the various sites described above, through several different mechanisms. At the spinal level, opioid-receptor stimulation inhibits the release of neurotransmitters. Thus the ability of a patient to recognize noxious peripheral stimulation is blunted. The mechanism underlying the supraspinal effects of morphine is less well understood, but there appear to be multiple foci of action.

As with benzodiazepines, the most significant deleterious side-effects of narcotics are related to the respiratory tract. Narcotics cause depressed function of the pontomedullary respiratory centers.[38] At low doses there is only a decrease in respiratory rate. However, as the dose increases, both rate and tidal volume decrease. This depression appears to occur earlier and to a greater degree in relation to the hypercapnic chemoreceptors compared to the hypoxic receptors. Thus even in the face of normal or near-normal oxygen saturation, the patient may be suffering from high serum CO_2 tension, due to decreased ventilation. This potential complication is particularly important in chronic obstructive pulmonary disease (COPD) patients, who have a pre-existing depressed hypoxic ventilatory drive. These respiratory depressive effects of narcotics are potentiated when the drugs are administered in conjunction with benzodiazepines. Narcotics can also produce a unique respiratory side-effect, due to their ability to cause endogenous histamine release. This increased serum histamine concentration may lead to H_1 agonism on bronchial smooth muscle, and consequent bronchospasm.

Narcotics also cause mild cardiovascular depression, mostly due to blunted baroreceptor reflexes and peripheral vasodilatation, which leads to systemic hypotension. This effect can be partially reversed by administration of antihistamines, suggesting that the histamine release caused by narcotics also plays a role in the cardiovascular side-effects. Narcotics also have a slight direct negative inotropic effect on the myocardium.

The gastrointestinal tract contains the second-highest number of opioid receptors. Systemic narcotics can cause several hazardous GI side-effects due to agonism at these mu-2-receptors. Initially, the overall resting tone of GI-tract smooth muscle is slightly increased, but eventually this is replaced by hypotonia or atony. There is also a decrease in the frequency and effectiveness of rhythmic, propulsive peristaltic waves. This effect is particularly important in patients on long-term narcotics (e.g. intensive-care unit (ICU) patients, chronic pain patients), who may develop obstructive constipation. Special consideration must also be given to patients with active ulcerative colitis, in whom the bowel stasis and atony may lead to bowel distension and the development of toxic megacolon.

Perhaps a more important potential GI complication is related to the effect of narcotics on the biliary system. Morphine causes constriction of the sphincter of

Oddi.[39] This may lead to markedly increased pressure in the common bile duct. Intracholecystic pressure can also be increased, inducing symptoms of biliary colic. These effects occur within minutes of intravenous injection, and can persist for several hours. This side-effect is of particular importance in patients with known obstructive biliary disease, and in those undergoing biliary interventional procedures.

With regard to clinical use, morphine and meperidine (Demerol®) play an important role as opiate narcotics for longer-term pain control, but have been largely replaced by fentanyl (Sublimaze®) and its congeners, sufentanil (Sufenta®) and alfentanil (Alfenta®), for systemic analgesia during percutaneous interventional procedures. One reason for this transition is the increased lipophilicity of these agents (fentanyl is 7000 times more lipophilic than morphine). This leads to much more rapid penetration into the CNS, more rapid onset of action, and thus more reliable and more reproducible analgesia. Morphine is metabolized in the liver by conjugation with glucuronic acid. One of the products of this metabolism is morphine-6-glucuronide. Compared to morphine, this metabolite is both more potent and has a longer effective half-life. This makes accurate titration for the desired analgesic effect much more difficult without introducing an increased risk of hazardous side-effects. A metabolite of meperidine, nor-meperidine, has been shown to cause tremors and seizures.[40] Fentanyl and its congeners have much shorter effective half-lives than morphine or meperidine, and have little significant effect from persisting active metabolites, allowing excellent titration of analgesia. In addition, fentanyl causes less spasm of the sphincter of Oddi and less nausea and vomiting than is commonly observed with morphine. Finally, fentanyl and its congeners cause little if any histamine release, and are thus preferred for patients with known reactive airway disease or hypotension. Only minimal cardiovascular depression is observed with fentanyl, even at high doses. However, it can cause slight bradycardia due to increased vagal tone. An unusual chest-wall rigidity can be seen with rapid injections of high doses of fentanyl. This appears to be due to stimulation of the spinal inspiratory motor neurons, creating a sustained inspiration that may lead to respiratory compromise.[41]

Reversal agents (Table 7.5)
Despite every attempt to titrate correctly the appropriate amounts of sedative and analgesic agents, unwanted side-effects will intermittently occur. The radiologist must be familiar with recognition and treatment of the hazardous side-effects.

There are two distinct pharmacologic reversal agents, one of which is effective for narcotic toxicity and the other for benzodiazepines. Specifically, naloxone (Narcan®) is an effective narcotic antagonist, while the antagonist effect of flumazenil (Romazicon®) is specifically directed against benzodiazepines.[5,42] The difficulty lies in distinguishing between a narcotic and a benzodiazepine overdose, which is complicated by the fact that the two drug classes produce similar complications. The correct decision is often dependent on close patient monitoring and documentation of the pharmacologic interventions employed during the procedure. This will be addressed more specifically later in this chapter.

Table 7.5 Reversal agents

Drug	Initial dose	Maximum dose	Onset of action
Naloxone[a]	0.1–0.2 mg	Titrate slowly	1–2 min
Nalmefene[a]	0.5–1 µg/kg	Titrate slowly	3–5 min
Flumazenil[b]	0.2–0.3 mg	3 mg/h	1–2 min

The doses listed are suggested when the agent is given alone to a healthy patient. Doses must be modified when used in combination and in patients with relevant comorbidity.

For all of the agents discussed, the package insert should be consulted for a full description of the doses, pharmacokinetics and contraindications.

[a]Used for reversal of opiates/opioids.
[b]Used for reversal of benzodiazepines.

Both flumazenil and naloxone are effective antagonists, but they also suffer from several limitations and potential hazards that must be emphasized. Both agents are very fast acting and produce notable clinical effects upon initial IV bolus. However, the effective half-lives of flumazenil and naloxone are shorter than those of their corresponding agonists. Thus it is not uncommon for patients to suffer a sedation or analgesic relapse following an appropriate initial response to a single dose of the reversal agent. The radiology team must therefore maintain vigilance in patient monitoring, and use repeated doses of reversal agents, as necessary. A new narcotic antagonist, nalmefene (Revex®), is similar to naloxone, but has a more prolonged duration of effect and may be useful in some situations. Finally, delivery of these reversal agents must be undertaken slowly and carefully. Rapid bolus administration can lead to heightened excitatory emergence effects, including nausea, vomiting, cardiac ectopy, tachycardia and seizures.[43]

Preprocedural evaluation

The responsibility for patient care immediately before, during and after the procedure lies with the radiologist. Thus it is incumbent on him or her to be familiar with the current state of health and past medical history of each patient, as these pertain to the intended procedure.

Preprocedural patient assessment is mandatory when the use of any type of sedation or analgesia is anticipated. This is best achieved by direct contact between the patient and the radiologist involved. As an alternative, the patient can be contacted by a nurse or other trained assistant. A screening questionnaire can help to ensure a complete assessment.

General patient status

The American Society of Anesthesiologists has developed a classification scheme (Table 7.6) that is used as an indicator of the degree of anesthetic risk and the expected frequency of post operative complications.[44] A similar scheme should be applied to prospective patients who are scheduled to undergo interventional procedures that will require conscious sedation. Level of baseline awareness or

Table 7.6 American Society of Anesthesiologists' (ASA) physical status classification[44]

ASA level	Description
I	Normal healthy patient
II	Patient with mild systemic disease
III	Patient with severe systemic disease
IV	Patient with severe systemic disease that is a constant threat to life
V	Moribund patient not expected to survive without operation

obtundation may also influence the degree of sedation that is considered to be safe, and may also serve as a reference point for the level of pharmacologically induced sedation.

The impact of advanced age must not be underestimated. This is becoming increasingly important as our population ages. In 1988, 12.3 per cent of the population in the USA was over 65 years old,[45] and this figure is projected to double by the year 2025. Certainly as the population ages and more percutaneous techniques are developed or refined, the number of interventions will increase dramatically. As patients age, several anatomic and physiologic changes occur. While these changes are considered 'normal' or expected, they nevertheless affect how patients tolerate conscious sedation and the stresses imposed by interventions. An excellent and comprehensive review article by Cheng describes the physiologic changes observed with aging and how these affect preoperative anesthetic evaluation.[46] His findings are germane to radiologists since, once again, conscious sedation is simply a less profound level along the continuous spectrum to general anesthesia. As expected, pulmonary, cardiovascular and renal disease are the primary causes of postoperative complications in older patients.[47] Thus the need to pay attention to pre-existing disease in these systems should be emphasized in the preprocedural evaluation.

Medical history

Perhaps the most important focus when obtaining a medical history is the evaluation of the appropriateness of performing the requested procedure. All interventional procedures involve inherent risks to the patient, and the radiologist must be able to defend confidently his or her decision to proceed with the intervention. In addition, close attention must be paid to possible compromise of the pulmonary and cardiovascular systems, since the pharmacologic agents used may further depress the functions of theses systems. Hepatic and renal diseases are not typically exacerbated by the drugs, but instead decreased function of these systems may lead to unexpected potentiation of the hazardous side-effects of the sedative and analgesic agents. Finally, overall patient condition, including advanced age, must be considered prior to the administration of any drugs.

Since respiratory depression is the most likely complication of these pharmacologic agents, caution must be exercised in the case of patients with pulmonary compromise. In lieu of the usual benzodiazepine-narcotic combination, perhaps a narcotic could be administered alone. Such patients will lose the anxiolysis and amnesia of the benzodiazepine, but will retain the sedation and, most importantly, the systemic analgesia provided by the narcotic. These patients could also have the benzodiazepine given early (i.e. immediately following preprocedural discussion with the radiologist) for anxiolysis. The analgesic could then be held until just prior to the first needle puncture. The drawback of this method is the requirement for patient monitoring over a longer period of time prior to initiation of the procedure. Another option is combining an antihistamine with an opioid. Antihistamines, like benzodiazepines, provide sedation as well as mild anxiolysis and amnesia. An antihistamine-narcotic combination would have less central respiratory depressive effect than would an equisedative benzodiazepine-narcotic dose. The choice of an antihistamine in lieu of a benzodiazepine may also be useful in patients with reactive airways disease, since the antihistamine may protect against the histamine release induced by the narcotic. However, patients with obstructive pulmonary disease should not be given antihistamines, as this will lead to thickening of bronchial secretions and a clinical exacerbation of their disease.

A history of cardiovascular disease should also influence decisions regarding sedation and analgesia, due to the depressive effects on the cardiovascular system exerted by the usual pharmacologic agents. Goldman et al. evaluated multiple cardiac risk factors in patients undergoing general anesthesia.[48] Those factors that were found to be associated with a significantly increased risk of intra-operative or postoperative cardiac complications included a history of myocardial infarction within the last 6 months, congestive heart failure, ectopic beats or non-sinus cardiac rhythm. Since conscious sedation employed during interventional radiologic procedures is simply a less profound form of anesthesia, Goldman's cardiac risk factors should also be considered by radiologists. Manipulations of the pharmacologic regimen, similar to those employed in patients with respiratory compromise, could be used for these patients. Patients with well-controlled hypertension do not appear to be at a significantly higher risk of sedation-related complications. However, it has been noted that these patients can react to conscious sedation drugs with an acute, precipitous drop in blood pressure.[49] This creates a significant risk of ischemia to end-organs (e.g. kidneys, brain, heart) that may already be tenuously perfused.[50] Therefore, in hypertensive patients the induction of sedation must be performed with particular care.

Significant hepatobiliary disease is important for several reasons. Nearly all of the pharmacologic agents that are used for conscious sedation are metabolized in the liver. In most cases, once metabolized, these agents lose their effectiveness. In patients with hepatocellular disease, the drugs are metabolized less quickly, so their effective half-lives are increased. In these patients, similar induction doses should be used, but the time intervals between doses must be increased because the rate of degradation of these drugs is decreased. Following metabolic breakdown of these agents by the hepatocytes, the metabolites may be excreted via the biliary system. Due to the effects of biliary obstruction on hepatic function, drug activity will also be prolonged in patients with biliary obstruction. In these cases, like those with hepatocellular disease, the initial induction dose may be similar, but additional dose amounts should be decreased and the time interval between doses increased.

The major plasma proteins are albumin, globulin and fibrinogen. Of these, albumin is the primary protein involved in the binding of circulating agents. Essentially all albumin and fibrinogen are created in the liver, and patients with hepatocellular dysfunction often suffer from hypoalbuminemia. This is important in the context of drug dosing for conscious sedation. Upon IV injection, benzodiazepines become very highly protein bound (85–98 per cent). Protein binding of narcotics is more varied, but fentanyl and its congeners have high (80–92 per cent) protein binding in circulation. As is shown in Fig. 7.1, a drop in serum albumin will cause an increase in unbound 'effective' agent. This increase in effect becomes more profound as an agent's normal protein-binding percentage increases. Therefore, since all of the typical agents used in conscious sedation are highly protein bound, caution must be exercised when administering these drugs to patients with hypoalbuminemia. These patients require a decrease in both initial and subsequent doses, as well as an increase in the interval between additional doses.

The kidneys serve as the primary route of excretion of drug metabolites, so there may be persistence of these active metabolites in patients with renal disease. Thus initial doses may remain standard, but follow-up doses must be decreased, and the interval between doses must be increased. Moreover, patients with a protein-losing nephropathy may have hypoproteinemia. Dosing modifications in the setting of hypoproteinemia are described above. Patients with renal dysfunction are also prone to electrolyte imbalances. In particular, hypo- and hyperkalemia can lead to myocardial irritability with a markedly increased risk of dysrhythmias during the emotional and physiologic stress of an interventional procedure.

Pharmacological history

It is important to know the patient's current medications, as they may affect the patient's response to conscious sedation or intervention, they may confuse the evaluation of suspected complications of the sedation or procedure, or they may even lead to catastrophic drug interactions.

Patients on anticoagulation therapy will be at increased risk of bleeding complications during the intervention. However, in some circumstances, an intervention is deemed necessary despite the presence of these agents, and these procedures must be performed with great care. There is a theoretical increased risk of bleeding in patients on aspirin or non-steroidal anti-inflammatory drugs (NSAIDs), but this has not been confirmed by clinical experience. Coumadin® (warfarin) is a vitamin K antagonist and thus inhibits the production of coagulation factors II, VII, IX and X, which are synthesized in the liver. The mean effective half-life of coumadin is approximately 40 h, with a duration of action of up to 4 days. The effects of coumadin can be reversed by the administration of vitamin K. Nevertheless, at least 24 h are still required to allow the generation of the necessary amounts of vitamin K-dependent coagulation factors. If this delay is considered to be unacceptable,

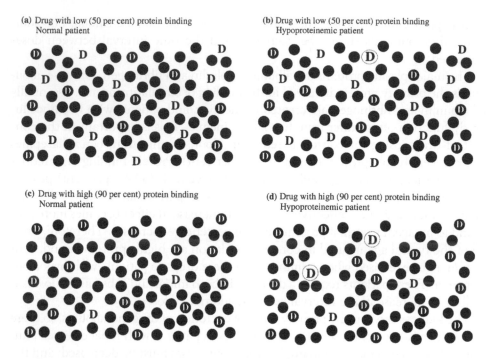

(a) Drug with low (50 per cent) protein binding
Normal patient

(b) Drug with low (50 per cent) protein binding
Hypoproteinemic patient

(c) Drug with high (90 per cent) protein binding
Normal patient

(d) Drug with high (90 per cent) protein binding
Hypoproteinemic patient

Figure 7.1 The circles represent plasma proteins, the letter 'D' within a circle represents bound drug, and the free letter 'D' represents unbound, active drug. In Figures 7.1b and d the letter 'D' with a surrounding dotted circle represents additional unbound, active drug released due to the hypoproteinemic state. (a) Presence of an intravenous agent, with a protein–binding level of 50 per cent, in a healthy patient; 10 of the 20 drug molecules (50 per cent) are unbound and produce the desired effects. If this same injected drug dose is given to a hypoproteinemic patient (b), one additional drug molecule will be unbound, increasing the effect of the drug on the patient by approximately 10 per cent. However, if the drug is normally highly protein bound (Figures 7.1c and d), the increase in effective dose is marked. (c) Presence of an intravenous agent with a protein-binding level of 90 per cent in a healthy patient. In this case, two of the drug molecules (10 per cent) are unbound and produce the desired effect. If an identical dose is given to a hypoproteinemic patient, an additional two drug molecules will be unbound. This increases the effect of the injected dose by 100 per cent, and will probably lead to a clinical overdose.

intravenous administration of coagulation factors through a transfusion of fresh-frozen plasma is the most reliable and prompt method of coumadin reversal.

Heparin serves as a catalytic template for the thrombin–antithrombin reaction. It is a cofactor for antithrombin III, increasing the reaction rate 1000-fold.[51] Heparin inhibits several additional activated coagulation factors. Parenteral heparin is degraded and disappears from the blood via first-order kinetics, and its effective half-life, while short (usually 1–2 h), is dependent on the dose administered. The anticoagulant effect typically disappears 2–8 h after discontinuation of heparin administration.[52] If this short resolution time is considered excessive, heparin's effects can be reversed with protamine. However, protamine has the potential side-effects of dyspnea, bradycardia, hypotension and, most importantly, anaphylaxis (particularly in diabetic patients who have used neutral protamine, Hagedorn (NPH) insulin). Protamine should therefore only be used in extreme circumstances, when waiting for heparin degradation is considered hazardous to the patient. Heparin allergies, which are relatively common, are another potential concern.

Salicylates and NSAIDs block the production of thromboxane A_2, which normally induces platelet aggregation and thrombosis.[51] The platelet dysfunction is permanent throughout the 7–10-day life of the platelet. However, the clinical effect on coagulation is generally minor, and for most vascular interventional procedures aspirin is prescribed. Nevertheless, if a procedure has a high risk of uncontrolled bleeding (e.g. large-core biopsy of a hypervascular mass), the effects of salicylates and NSAIDs can be reversed by transfusion of fresh, unaffected platelets.

Patients who are on CNS depressants will experience much more profound sedation following the administration of procedural pharmacologic agents. Since much of the respiratory and cardiovascular depression caused by sedative and analgesic agents is due to effects on the brainstem, these complications will be much more frequent and profound in patients who are already receiving CNS depressants.

The presence of beta-blockers can lead to a misleading response in the face of hypotension, which may be a consequence of either excessive sedation or a procedure-related complication. Due to the depression of cardiac chronotropy by the beta-blocking agent, the patient will not react to hypotension with the necessary and expected tachycardia. Instead, such patients appear to be suffering from a vasovagal reaction (i.e. hypotension and bradycardia). Consequently, without pre-procedural knowledge of the beta-blocker, the radiologist may erroneously conclude that atropine is necessary. Instead, these patients may require epinephrine or a selective beta-agonist, such as isoproterenol (Isuprel®).

Special mention must be made of monoamine oxidase (MAO) inhibitors. These agents are antidepressants that are often used when tricyclic antidepressants are clinically ineffective. Fortunately, their use has decreased significantly, especially in the USA. An idiopathic toxic interaction can occur when certain narcotics are used in a patient who is on MAO inhibitors, precipitating severe and often lethal hypertension and hyperthemia.[53] If an interventional procedure is deemed necessary, narcotics should be avoided or, conversely, patients should be taken off their MAO inhibitors for at least 14 days prior to the procedure.

Physical examination

A brief, directed physical examination of the patient should be performed prior to the procedure. In general, heart rate, blood pressure and respiratory rate should be measured and recorded, mainly in order to serve as reference points during the procedure. Inspection of the prospective site of intervention should also be carried out as part of preprocedural planning to ensure a safe, clean skin intervention site. In patients undergoing angiographic procedures, peripheral pulses should be measured and recorded both before and after the procedure.

Following review of the patient's history and a focused physical examination, the radiologist should preview the procedural steps with the patient. It is also necessary to discuss other diagnostic options and potential complications of the procedure. Informed consent should also be obtained from the patient or a selected family member after questions and concerns have been addressed. During this meeting it is critical that the radiologist be genuine, competent and caring. The value of gaining the patient's confidence cannot be underestimated. A recent study by Egbert showed that a preoperative visit and discussion between the anesthesiologist and the patient had a considerable calming effect.[54] In fact, this meeting was equivalent in effectiveness to a dose of preoperative barbiturate in achieving patient compliance and ease of induction of anesthesia.[54] A similar phenomenon can be expected to occur when a trusting doctor–patient relationship is established prior to radiologic procedures.

Legal concerns are always involved in the performance of an examination. The outcome of legal action depends not only on the laws and interpretations in that particular jurisdiction, and the empiric definition of 'usual and customary practice', but also on communication, primarily between the patient and physician. Most claims in radiology relate to either misdiagnoses or missed diagnoses. Even in interventional radiology, relatively few claims relate specifically to the performance of the procedure, outcomes of a procedure or complications of ancillary medications.

Informed consent is often seen as a major concern. There are a number of relevant principles in relation to informed consent. First, the standards for informed consent vary, to a certain extent, according to jurisdiction and state. If informed consent is obtained, certain states mandate that the patient be informed only of what a reasonable physician would think is relevant to the examination. However, an increasing number of states utilize the 'reasonable patient' standard, requiring that the patient must be told what a 'reasonable patient' would want to know in similar circumstances. Secondly, informed consent must be individualized. If informed consent is to be obtained, it is not sufficient to utilize one preprinted sheet for all patients in all situations. The specific risks for any given patient must be elucidated. This does not mean that a standardized information sheet cannot be used, but the patient must be given the opportunity to discuss any specific examination or procedure with the physician, assuming that the patient wants to do so, and that a significant risk exists.

The question of when informed consent is necessary is a difficult one. As a basic guide, informed consent should be obtained whenever significant risk to the patient exists. Thus informed consent is not necessary for a chest X-ray or for a CT scan without contrast, but clearly it is necessary for a situation in which medications, such as sedatives, will be utilized, or for any interventional procedure. A basic principle to keep in mind with regard to informed consent is that if the patient consents to a substantial risk, he or she is in essence consenting to a lesser risk. For example, if a patient is informed that a particular medication involves a small risk of death or stroke, and the patient consents to its use, he or she is giving implied consent to less substantial risks such as bronchospasm or severe urticaria.

Procedural monitoring

As the patient arrives in the radiology suite, several preparatory steps, which have been previously discussed, have been accomplished. Both the patient and the attending radiology assistants should have a good understanding of the proposed procedure. Baseline vital signs have been acquired and recorded on a permanent form which can serve as a reference point during procedural monitoring. This form is also best used for continued documentation of procedural detail and postprocedural care. Teamwork, while necessary in all phases of the patient's care, is particularly significant during the procedure itself, when the radiologist's attention is intensively directed towards the technical details of the actual procedure. Consequently, the designated radiology nurse or technologist becomes 'the eyes and ears' of the radiologist and assumes a central role in the delivery of care and comfort to the patient.

It should be stressed that the need for and degree of conscious sedation should never be regarded as routine. A recent survey of 634 members of the Society of Cardiovascular and Interventional Radiology described a broad range of levels of sedation used, and also revealed some trends that may serve as guidelines.[55] In general, diagnostic procedures require less time and, therefore, less sedation. Therapeutic procedures, especially those involving solid organs (e.g. biliary interventions, transjugular intrahepatic portosystemic (TIPS) shunt procedures, nephrostomy/stent placements) require more time and catheter manipulation, and thus require more profound sedation. Another important trend revealed in this study was that procedures involving the thorax were typically performed with very light sedation. This is probably partly due to the increased risk of respiratory compromise in these patients and also to the brief nature of the intervention.

Routine patient monitoring

Both the Joint Commission for Accreditation of Healthcare Organizations (JCAHO) and the American Society of Anesthesiologists (ASA) consider conscious sedation to be a form of anesthesia, due to the potential loss of protective reflexes associated with sedating agents.[56] Thus strict attention needs to be paid to patient monitoring. Open communication is important, since it not only comforts the patient, but probably also promotes greater trust and confidence in the patient. This improves patient compliance and increases the likelihood of technical success. It is also likely to enable earlier recognition and more accurate characterization of procedural or drug-related complications.

A list of routine monitoring equipment is shown in Table 7.7. All patients should have a functioning IV line in place, whether or not IV conscious sedation is planned. Since procedural complications are never planned and nearly always require IV access, it is safest to have access immediately available. Patients who are receiving conscious sedation should also have an automated blood-pressure cuff and pulse oximeter placed. Readings should be recorded every 5–10 mins in the patient record. Respiratory rate and heart rate should also be measured and recorded at the same intervals.

Table 7.7   Monitoring equipment for routine sedation

- Automated blood-pressure cuff
- Pulse oximeter
- IV equipment (needles, tubing, fluid)
- ECG monitor
- Oxygen source
- Oxygen delivery devices (nasal cannula, partial non-rebreathing mask)

The most common complication of sedation or analgesic agents is respiratory depression. In addition, the cardiac dysrhythmias associated with sedation most commonly occur during periods of oxygen desaturation.[57] Thus the subject of pulse oximetry deserves special attention. Since the introduction of pulse oximetry in the 1980s, its use has increased rapidly.[58] Pulse oximetry functions by emitting light at wavelengths that are sensitive to oxyhemoglobin. Changes in the amount of light absorption measured by a microprocessor provide an estimate of percentage arterial oxygen saturation (SaO_2) of hemoglobin.[59] Although modern pulse oximetry devices have excellent accuracy, several caveats regarding knowledgeable use and interpretation of their results must be emphasized.

Since the pulse oximeter is measuring only SaO_2, the partial pressure of carbon dioxide (PCO_2) is unknown. The PCO_2 can vary widely and change independently of the partial pressure of oxygen (PO_2). Thus a patient may have a normal SaO_2 pulse-oximeter reading and still have a dangerously elevated PCO_2. Frumin et al., using experimental methods of apneic oxygenation,[60] were able to elevate PCO_2 up to 250 mmHg (normal range = 40–60 mmHg) and consequently drop blood pH to 6.72 (normal value = 7.4). During this interval of marked hypercapnia, the recorded SaO_2 was never below 98 per cent. Anesthesia and death can result from PCO_2 levels above 150 mmHg. This emphasizes the potential for dissociation of hypoxia and hypercapnia. The degree of retained CO_2 is based almost exclusively on the rate and depth of ventilation. Greater ventilation allows reduction of PCO_2. Thus, even patients with normal SaO_2 readings during a procedure must be reminded by the radiology team to make continual deep ventilatory efforts in order to ensure normal levels of blood CO_2.

The second point regarding appropriate use of the pulse oximeter is based on the relationship between SaO_2 and PO_2. The sigmoid shape of the oxygen saturation curve is generated by the nonlinear saturation and desaturation of the hemoglobin molecule with oxygen (Fig. 7.2). Since successful human aerobic life exists along the toe of this curve, SaO_2 readings from a pulse oximeter can lead to errant complacency on the part of the unfamiliar user. At the toe of the curve, very large changes in PO_2 (along the x-axis of Fig. 7.2) cause only very slight changes in SaO_2 (along the y-axis of Fig. 7.2). Since the radiologist is seeing only the SaO_2 reading, he or she must understand that slight drops in the pulse-oximeter reading may in fact reflect significant and dangerous drops in PO_2. Any reading at or below 90 per cent SaO_2 (equivalent to a PO_2 of 60 mmHg) must be regarded as hypoxemia. At 85 per cent SaO_2,

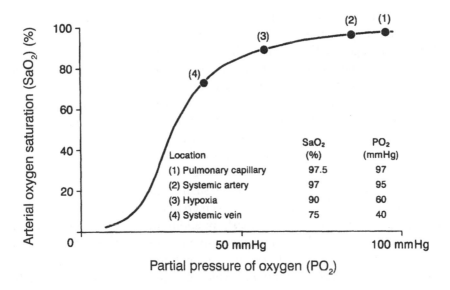

Figure 7.2   The graph shows the normal sigmoid shape of the oxygen saturation curve, with several specific points listed on the inset table. It is important to note the very minimal positive slope ($^x/_y$) at the toe (upper-right portion) of the curve. As a consequence of this minimal slope, very large changes in the partial pressure of oxygen (PO_2) are reflected on the pulse oximeter as very minimal changes in the percentage saturation (SaO_2). For example, a 0.5 per cent drop in SaO_2 from point 1 to point 2 reflects a 2-mmHg drop in PO_2. Moving from point 1 to point 3 would be seen as only a 7.5 per cent drop in SaO_2, but this 'slight' drop seen on the pulse oximeter would reflect a drop in PO_2 of 37 mmHg (a 'significant' 38 per cent drop in the patient's PO_2). Thus it must be emphasized that slight changes in what the radiology team sees on the pulse oximeter may actually reflect much more dramatic drops in the patient's partial oxygen pressure.

the patient's respiratory status is at the steep part of the desaturation curve, heading towards respiratory crisis. Ideally, the patient's ventilation and oxygenation should be corrected long before that level is reached. Patients with COPD must be very carefully observed in this context. They often have a baseline SaO_2 of 90–92 per cent and may therefore be significantly endangered with minimal sedation.

The routine use of ECG monitors and supplementary oxygen in young, asymptomatic healthy patients remains the subject of debate, and therefore policies should be developed for each institution. Certainly all patients with a history of pulmonary or cardiovascular disease should have cardiac monitoring and be given supplementary oxygen. The same could be said for patients undergoing prolonged procedures or ones expected to be especially painful, and for those who may need a deeper level of sedation.

Patient monitoring during complications

Complications that occur during an interventional radiologic procedure may be due to the pharmacologic agents used, procedure-related injury or underlying disease processes. Drug-related complications are usually due to overdosing. Another important but less often addressed complication is the underutilization of sedative and anesthetic agents. This leads to the 'complication' of unnecessary patient suffering. This may be due to a lack of familiarity with the drugs and a consequent timidity in seeking to achieve appropriate and adequate effects of these agents. Providing effective pharmacological protection for the interventional patient is a necessary skill for those who choose to perform interventional procedures, and this requires a personal interest on the part of the radiologist.

The two most common side-effects of overdosing are respiratory depression and hypotension. Recognition of respiratory depression is based on detection of either a low SaO_2 or a drop in respiratory rate. Usually one or both of these can be successfully resolved by the addition of supplementary oxygen either via a nasal cannula[61] or a partial non-rebreathing mask. In addition, attempts should be made to coach the patient to make several successive deep respiratory efforts. Although hypoxemia and even apnea do occur, most patients can be aroused easily and instructed to force deep ventilation,[11] which will usually overcome the deficit. If hypoxemia persists and drug overdose is still suspected, a reversal agent can be given to help to overcome the side-effects of either the benzodiazepine (using flumazenil) or the narcotic (using naloxone), or both. As stated earlier, care must be exercised to avoid administering these agents too quickly, as hazardous excitatory complications can occur upon patient emergence. If supplementary oxygenation and drug reversal are unsuccessful, a procedural complication (e.g. pneumothorax, hemorrhage) should be considered. These patients will typically indicate pain that may suggest these complications as the cause. Further imaging will often confirm the presence of these procedure-related injuries. Other complications that may lead to respiratory difficulties include an acute myocardial infarction or cerebrovascular accident.

Should respiratory compromise persist despite the above measures, assisted ventilation is necessary. Of the methods listed in Table 7.8, the need for use of a bag-valve mask (Ambu-bag®), with or without a nasopharyngeal or oropharyngeal airway, should be stressed. This combination should be regarded as the first and perhaps only line of intervention by a radiologist for providing assisted ventilation. Nasopharyngeal airways should be used in conscious patients who will not tolerate the oropharyngeal airway due to reflex gagging. Following placement, as necessary, of either of the airways, the bag-valve-mask can be successfully used with little training or practice. This method allows delivery of a very high percentage of oxygen, sufficient to oxygenate the patient while awaiting the Code team.

Placement of an endotracheal (ET) tube is also an effective method of assisting ventilation and supplying high levels of oxygen. The inflatable cuff of the ET tube has the added advantage of protecting the airway from aspiration of gastric contents, which is not possible with the Ambu-bag® setup. Nevertheless, in contradistinction to the Ambu-bag, use of a laryngoscope and successful placement of an appropriate ET tube require a great deal of skill and familiarity with the technique. Although many radiologists may have some degree of competency in its use, most

Table 7.8 Monitoring equipment necessary to address complications

- All equipment from Table 7.7
- Stethoscope
- Suction equipment
- Ambu-bag with facemask
- Nasopharyngeal and oropharyngeal airway devices
- Laryngoscope and endotracheal tubes
- Crash cart containing appropriate pharmacologic agents
- Defibrillator

do not. The consequences of unsuccessful ET tube placement in an emergent setting can be hazardous or even lethal to the patient. In general, ET tube placement should be performed only by specially trained personnel. Radiologists should focus their respiratory resuscitation efforts on the use of the simpler, but very effective, bag-valve mask.

Hypotension is the second most common complication and, like respiratory depression, may also be due to either sedative-analgesic drugs or the procedure itself. Early or mild hypotension can typically be treated with an increase in the rate of IV fluid administration. If a procedure-related hemorrhage is suspected (e.g. the procedure involves a highly vascular organ or tumor, or the patient is complaining of new unexpected pain or pressure), further imaging will often reveal a hemorrhage that may be the source of hypotension. Persistent hypotension may also be treated with various vasopressors (e.g. epinephrine, ephedrine or dopamine). Depending on the degree and rate of fall of the blood pressure, serial imaging, embolotherapy or surgical intervention should be considered. Vasovagal reactions are a third cause of hypotension, and should also always be considered in patients undergoing interventional procedures. Vasovagal reactions are not uncommon and should not be confused with a more typical hypotensive reaction due to hypovolemia. They are characterized by hypotension without reactive tachycardia or with bradycardia. This is an important distinction, since vasovagal reactions are best treated with atropine rather than vasopressors.

Immediately following the successful completion of a complication-free procedure, there is a natural tendency to decrease the level of attention given to the patient. However, increased vigilance, is necessary during the immediate postprocedural interval. During the procedure, the level of painful iatrogenic stimuli and degree of patient anxiety dictate the amount of sedative-analgesic administered. While the amounts of pharmacologic agents may be perfectly titrated during the painful procedure, this appropriate dose may have the effect of an overdose when the noxious stimuli have been removed. Thus, immediately following completion of the procedure, the radiology team should be prepared to address clinical changes that suggest a drug overdose.

Routine procedural documentation is modified when a complication occurs. The timing, treatment and outcome must all be documented. Monitoring of vital signs should be tailored to each specific situation. All pharmacologic or other interventions, as well as the patient's response to these, should be accurately recorded. This information is critical for appropriate continued monitoring and corrective intervention during the postprocedural period.

Postprocedural care and discharge

Following completion of the interventional procedure and stabilization of any complications, all patients should be observed. This observation is best carried out in a specialized room that is staffed by a member of the radiology team, a radiology nurse or a nurse anesthetist. As in the procedure room, appropriate and similar monitoring equipment (see Tables 7.7 and 7.8) should be available. When the patient is brought to the postprocedure room, the radiology team member should present the patient to the attending observation personnel. This presentation should include a description of the procedure and the types and amounts of sedative-analgesic agents used, any complications suffered, and treatment actions taken in order to address complications. In addition to this verbal presentation, the written documentation can be given to the observation staff and used for continued documentation of postprocedural monitoring.

During this period, the patient's vital signs are measured and recorded. The time interval between these measurements can be slowly increased if the patient remains clinically stable. The patient's increasing level of arousal may lead to new complaints that were not previously voiced due to the effects of the pharmacologic agents. Once the patient is well oriented and their vital signs and clinical signs and symptoms have remained normal, the patient should be discharged from the radiology department. Formal requirements for discharge (see example shown in Table 7.9) should be developed for each institution, and these criteria should be met by all patients who are leaving the hospital.

Prior to discharge, a final written assessment should be made by the radiologist or assistant. This should address the stability of the vital signs and the patient's final overall disposition. A radiology team member should also explain follow-up care to the patient. It is important to include a family member in this discussion, since the patient may still have some residual sedation or amnesia as a consequence of the medications given. This meeting also serves as a final opportunity for the radiologist to address any further concerns or questions that the patient or family may have. For outpatients, a set of written follow-up instructions should be given to the patient for future reference. This should include a point of contact to be used should the patient suffer a delayed complication. For inpatients, follow-up care instructions can be written into the hospital notes to direct the primary physician.

Conclusion

The specialty of diagnostic radiology has grown significantly in its capacities, and has benefited from the development of many new imaging techniques and, perhaps

Table 7.9 Discharge criteria

- Return to baseline vital signs (stable for 30–60 min)
- No orthostasis
- Intact, oriented mental status
- Ability to tolerate oral intake
- Ability to urinate
- Responsible adult in attendance

---

even more dramatically, new interventional techniques. A recent report by Drucker calculated a two to threefold increase in peripheral angioplasty procedures alone from 1989 to 1992.[62] Certainly a similar increase appears to have occurred in the performance of other radiological interventional procedures.

While the practice of radiology has been a beneficiary of this trend, perhaps the more important benefits have been extended to our patients. With few exceptions, imaging-guided procedures are less expensive, less invasive and less morbid than the corresponding surgical procedures. However, the continued provision of excellent radiological care is based on the premise that radiologists are performing these tasks with the appropriate technique. It must be emphasized that successful technique involves more than simply performing the intervention itself correctly.

In this arena of interventional procedural medicine, the breadth of responsibility borne by the radiologist is increased. A primary responsibility of all healthcare providers is to minimize or prevent the suffering of the patients in their care. During interventional radiologic procedures, the main components of patient comfort include anxiolysis, sedation, analgesia and amnesia. These four characteristics of patient comfort in interventional radiology are the same as those provided by anesthesiologists during general anesthesia, but are simply applied at less profound levels of depression. The JCAHO mandates that, 'in the interests of assuring patient and staff safety, training programs, policies and procedures, and monitoring systems should be in place whenever anesthesia is used within the hospital'.[56]

A report published in 1990 revealed that 86 deaths related to the use of midazolam had been reported to the Department of Health and Human Services.[11] Of these, 83 deaths (96 per cent) had occurred outside the operating-room setting, where the level of familiarity and standards for assessment and care are less well defined. Thus all radiologists who choose to participate in the performance of sedation-assisted procedures obligate themselves to a full understanding of the preprocedural workup, procedural monitoring techniques, postprocedural care and use of various pharmacologic agents to ensure patient comfort. An important aspect of this obligation lies in the training of allied personnel. Teamwork is essential during these procedures, requiring excellent, reliable nursing and technical support staff to work alongside the radiologist who is performing the procedure. A high level of continued physician and staff education and awareness will ensure that our patients receive appropriate, safe and comfortable care while they are in the radiology department.

References

1. Holzman RS, Cullen DJ, Eichhorn JH et al. Guidelines for sedation by nonanesthesiologists during diagnostic and therapeutic procedures. *Journal of Clinical Anesthesia* 1994; **6**: 265–76.

2. Mackenzie N, Grant IS. Comparison of propofol with methohexitone in the provision of anaesthesia for surgery under regional blockade. *British Journal of Anaesthesia* 1985; **57**: 1167–72.

3. Randall LO, Schallek W, Heise GA et al. The psychoactive properties of methaminodiazepoxide. *Journal of Pharmacology and Experimental Therapeutics* 1960; **129**: 163.

4. Martin IL. The benzodiazepines and their receptors: 25 years of progress. *Neuropharmacology* 1987; **26**: 957–70.

5. Salomen MA, Maze M. Molecular mechanism of action for hypnotic and sedative agents. In: Feldman SA, Paton W, Scurr C, eds. *Mechanisms of drugs in anesthesia*, 2nd edn. London: Hodder and Stoughton Ltd, 1993: 201–11.

6. Rall TW. Hypnotics and sedatives; ethanol. In: Gilman AG, Rall TW, Nies AS, Taylor P, eds. *The pharmacological basis of theraputics*, 8th edn. New York: Pergamon Press, 1990: 345–82.

7. Finder RL, Moore PA, Close JM. Flumazenil reversal of conscious sedation induced with intravenous fentanyl and diazepam. *Anaethesia Progress* 1995; **42**: 11–16.

8. Ghoneim MM, Mewaldt SP. Benzodiazepines and human memory: a review. *Anesthesiology* 1990; **72**: 926–38.

9. Stoelting RK. Benzodiazepines. In: *Pharmacology and physiology in anesthetic practice*, 1st edn. Philadelphia, PA: J.B. Lippincott, 1987: 118–31.

10. Alexander CM, Gross J. Sedative doses of midazolam depress hypoxic ventilatory responses in humans. *Anesthesia and Analgesia* 1988; **67**: 377–82.

11. Bailey PL, Pace NL, Ashburn MA et al. Frequent hypoxemia and apnea after sedation with midazolam and fentanyl. *Anesthesiology* 1990; **73**: 826–30.

12. Rao S, Sherbaniuk R, Prasad RW et al. Cardiopulmonary effects of diazepam. *Clinical Pharmacology and Therapeutics* 1973; **14**: 182–9.

13. Dundee JW, Halliday NJ, Loughran PG et al. The influence of age on the onset of anaesthesia with midazolam. *Anaesthesia* 1985; **40**: 441.

14. Whitwarm JG, Al Khudhairi D, McCloy RF. Comparison of midazolam and diazepam in doses of comparable potency during gastroscopy. *British Journal of Anaesthesia* 1983; **55**: 773–7.

15. Barker I, Butchart DGM, Gibson J et al. IV sedation for conservative dentistry. A comparison of midazolam and diazepam. *British Journal of Anaesthesia* 1986; **58**: 371–7.

16. Yamashiro M. Effectiveness of conscious sedation with a single benzodiazepine compared with a combination of drugs. *Anesthesia Progress* 1995; **42**: 103–6.

17. Arendt RM, Greenblatt DJ, deJong RH et al. *In vivo* correlates of benzodiazepine cerebrospinal fluid uptake, pharmacodynamic action and peripheral distribution. *Journal of Pharmacology and Experimental Therapeutics* 1983; **227**: 98.

18. McNeir DA, Mainous EG, Tieger N. Propofol as an intravenous agent in general anesthesia and conscious sedation. *Anesthesia Progress* 1988; **35**: 147–51.

19. Mirakhur RK. Induction characteristics of propofol in children: comparison with thiopentone. *Anesthesiology* 1988; **43**: 593–8.

20. Snellen F, Lauwers P, Demeyere R et al. The use of midazolam versus propofol for short-term sedation following coronary artery bypass grafting. *Intensive Care Medicine* 1990; **16**: 312–16.

21. Higgins TL, Yared JP, Estafanous FG et al. Propofol versus midazolam for intensive-care unit sedation after coronary artery bypass grafting. *Critical Care Medicine* 1994; **22**: 1415–23.

22. Manninen PH, Chan ASH, Papworth D. Conscious sedation for interventional neuroradiology: a comparison of midazolam and propofol infusions. *Canadian Journal of Anaesthesia* 1997; **44**: 26–30.

23. Valtonen M, Lisalo E, Kanto J et al. Propofol as an induction agent in children: pain on injection and pharmacokinetics. *Acta Anaesthesiologica Scandinavica* 1989; **33**: 152–5.

24. Garrison JC. Histamine, bradykinin, 5-hydroxytryptamine, and their antagonists. In: Gillman AG, Rall TW, Nies AS, Taylor P, eds. *The pharmacologic basis of therapeutics*, 8th edn. New York: Pergamon Press, 1990: 575–99.

25. Ritchie JM, Greene NM. Local anesthetics. In Gillman AG, Rall TW, Nies AS, Taylor P, eds. *The pharmacologic basis of therapeutics*, 8th edn. New York: Pergamon Press, 1990: 311–31.

26. Walters BL: Pain control in the emergency department. In Reisdorf EJ, Roberts MR, Wiegenstein JG, eds. *Pediatric emergency medicine*. Philadelphia, PA: W.B. Saunders & Co., 1993: 908–15.

27. Covino BG. Systemic toxicity of local anesthetic agents (editorial). *Anesthesia and Analgesia* 1978; **57**: 387.

28. Vandel KJ, Steiner JF. Administering local anesthetics safely, effectively and painlessly. *Journal of the American Academy of Physician Assistants* 1993; **6**: 581–7.

29. Covino BG. Toxicity and systemic effects of local anesthetic agents. In: Strichartz GR, ed. *Local anesthetics. Handbook of experimental pharmacology. Volume 81.* Berlin: Springer-Verlag, 1987; 187–212.

30. Doyle DJ. A closer look at local anesthetics. *Emergency Medicine* 1991; **23**: 147–52.

31. McKay W, Morris R, Mushlin P. Comparison of pain associated with intradermal and subcutaneous infiltration with various local anesthetic solutions. *Anesthesia and Analgesia* 1987; **66**: 1180–92.

32. Mader TJ, Playe SJ, Garb JL. Reducing the pain of local anesthetic infiltration: warming and buffering have a synergistic effect. *Annals of Emergency Medicine* 1994; **23**: 550–54.

33. Green SM, Rothrock SG, Gorchynski J. Validation of diphenhydramine as a dermal local anesthetic. *Annals of Emergency Medicine* 1994; **23**: 1284–9.

34. Jaffe JH, Martin WR. Opioid analgesics and antagonists. In: Gillman AG, Rall TW, Nies AS, Taylor P, eds. *The pharmacologic basis of therapeutics*, 8th edn. New York: Pergamon Press, 1990: 485–521.

35. Pert CB, Snyder SH. Opioid receptor: demonstrated in nervous tissue. *Science* 1973; **179**: 1011.

36. Simon EJ, Hiller JM, Edelman I. Stereospecific binding of the potent narcotic analgesic Hetorphine to rat brain homogenates. *Proceedings of the National Academy of Sciences of the USA* 1973; **70**: 1947–9.

37. Terenius L. Characteristics of the 'receptor' for narcotic analgesics in synaptic plasma membrane fractions from rat brain. *Acta Pharmacologica et Toxicologica* 1973; **33**: 377.

38. Buck ML, Blumer JL. Opioids and other analgesics. Adverse effects in the intensive-care unit. *Critical Care Clinics* 1991; **7**: 615.

39. Teeple E Jr. Pharmacology and physiology of narcotics. *Critical Care Clinics* 1990; **6**: 255.

40. Proudfoot J. Analgesia, anesthesia and conscious sedation. *Emergency Medicine Clinics of North America* 1995; **13**: 357–79.

41. Streisand JB, Bailey PH, LeMaire L *et al.* Fentanyl-induced rigidity and unconsciousness in human volunteers. *Anesthesiology* 1993; **78**: 4–10.

42. Gross JB, Blouin RT, Zandsberg S *et al.* Effect of flumazenil on ventilatory drive during sedation with midazolam and alfentanil. Anesthesiology 1996; **85**: 713–20.

43. Andree RA. Sudden death following naloxone administration. *Anaesthesia and Analgesia* 1980; **59**: 782–4.

44. Cohen MM, Duncan PG. Physical status score and trends in anesthetic complications. *Journal of Clinical Epidemiology* 1988; **41**: 83–90.

45. US Bureau of the Census. *Statistical abstracts of the United States* 1990, 110th edn. Washington, DC: US Bureau of the Census, 1990: 12.

46. Cheng EY, Wang-Cheng RM. Impact of aging on preoperative evaluation. *Journal of Clinical Anesthesia* 1991; **3**: 324–44.

47. Older P, Smith R. Experience with the preoperative invasive measurement of haemodynamic, respiratory and renal function in 100 elderly patients scheduled for major abdominal surgery. *Anaesthesia and Intensive Care* 1988; **16**: 389–95.

48. Goldman L, Caldera DL, Nussbaum SR *et al.* Multifactorial index of cardiac risk in noncardiac surgical procedures. *New England Journal of Medicine* 1977; **297**: 845–50

49. Harshfield DL, Teplick SK, Brandon JC. Pain control during interventional biliary procedures: epidural anesthesia vs. IV sedation. *American Journal of Roentgenology* 1993; **161**: 1057–9.

50. Brown BR Jr. Anesthesia for the patient with essential hypertension. *Seminars in Anesthesia* 1987; **6**: 79–92.

51. Majerus PW, Broze GJ, Miletich JP *et al.* Anticoagulant, thrombolytic and antiplatelet drugs. In: Gillman AG, Rall TW, Nies AS, Taylor P, eds. *The pharmacologic basis of therapeutics*, 8th edn. New York: Pergamon Press, 1990: 1311–31.

52. Weitz JI. Low-molecular-weight heparins. *New England Journal of Medicine* 1997; **337**: 688–98.

53. Baldessarini RJ. Drugs and the treatment of psychiatric disorders. In: Goodman-Gillman A, Rall TW, Nies AS, Taylor P, eds. *The pharmacologic basis of therapeutics*, 8th edn. New York: Pergamon Press, 1990: 383–435.

54. Egbert LD, Battit GE, Turndorf H, Beecher HK. The value of the pre-operative visit by an anesthetist. *Journal of the American Medical Association* 1963; **185**: 553–5.

55. Wittenberg KH, Mueller PR, Kaufman JA *et al.* Patterns of anesthesia and nursing care for interventional radiology procedures: a national survey of physician practices and preferences. *Radiology* 1997; **202**: 339–43.

56. Joint Commission on Accreditation of Healthcare Organizations. *Accreditation manual for hospitals*. Oakbrook Terrace, IL: Joint Commission on Accreditation of Healthcare Organizations, 1993.

57. Katz AS, Michelson EL, Stawicki J *et al.* Cardiac arrhythmias: frequency during fiberoptic bronchoscopy and correlation with hypoxemia. *Archives of Internal Medicine* 1981; **141**: 603–8.

58. Barker SJ, Tremper KK. Pulse oximetry: applications and limitations. *International Anaesthesiology Clinics* 1987; **25**: 155–75.

59. Kidd JF, Vickers MD. Pulse oximeters: essential monitors with limitations. *British Journal of Anaesthesia.* 1989; **62**: 355–7.

60. Frumin MJ, Epstein RM, Cohen G. Apneic oxygenation in man. *Anesthesiology* 1959; **20**: 789–98.

61. Bell GD, Morden A, Brown S *et al.* Prevention of hypoxemia during upper gastrointestinal endoscopy by means of oxygen via nasal cannula. *Lancet* 1987; **1**: 1022–4.

62. Drucker EA, Brennan TA. The turf war was over peripheral vascular intervention. I. Setting the stage. *Radiology* 1994; **193**: 81A–86A.

Pediatric conscious sedation

Jane S. Matsumoto and John T. Wald

Conscious sedation is defined as a state of depressed consciousness in which the patient can be aroused by verbal or physical stimuli, maintains protective airway reflexes, and independently maintains a patent airway. Deep sedation is defined as a state of depressed consciousness from which the patient is not easily aroused, and which may be accompanied by a partial or complete loss of protective reflexes and inability to maintain a patent airway independently. However, sedation is a dynamic state, and there is controversy over whether true 'conscious' sedation exists.[1,2] The level of consciousness may follow a continuum between conscious and deep sedation during a single sedation procedure. The potential for any sedation procedure to advance to unintended deep levels of sedation, with their attendant risks, mandates close vigilance, constant monitoring and continued reassessment of the sedated child.

Pediatric conscious sedation methods have developed in radiology to facilitate safe, high-quality diagnostic examinations on young or uncooperative children. The level of sedation required varies with the age of the patient and the type of examination requested. Magnetic resonance imaging (MRI) requires a longer period of sedation and less movement than most computed tomography (CT) examinations. Interventional procedures, by definition, are painful and require analgesia in addition to sedation. There is rarely a need for sedation for gastrointestinal (GI) fluoroscopy or voiding cystourethrography, and in fact, sedation may hinder such studies.

The increasing frequency of use of pediatric sedation for examinations and procedures throughout medicine prompted the American Academy of Pediatrics (AAP) to address this issue. In 1992, the AAP published *Guidelines for Monitoring and Management of Pediatric Patients, During and After Sedation for Diagnostic and Therapeutic Procedures*.[3] These guidelines give recommendations for pre- and post-procedure evaluation, monitoring, recovery, education, equipment, personnel and medication for sedation. The guidelines also emphasize the need for attendant medical personnel to be trained in sedation and monitoring techniques and airway management of children.

The Joint Commission on Accreditation of Healthcare Organizations has also begun to address the issue of conscious sedation standards, and they emphasize the establishment of conscious sedation guidelines in each medical institution, which need to be consistently followed, resulting in uniform standards of care.[4] Guidelines, education and competencies for physicians and nurses are being developed by medical institutions to ensure that conscious sedation procedures are being performed by trained and qualified personnel in a consistent manner.[5,6]

Presedation evaluation

It is helpful to contact the parent or caregiver one or more days in advance in order to determine whether the child needs sedation, whether there are contraindications to sedation, and to obtain a pertinent medical history. Infants less than 1 month old may not need sedation. If they are kept awake before the examination, fed and swaddled, they may fall asleep for the length of a noninvasive study such as a CT or MRI examination. If children will require sedation, it is often helpful to keep them up late the night before the study and to wake them early in the morning so that they are already sleepy before sedation is given.

The fasting policy should be explained to the parent or caregiver. The child should be fasting from solids for 4 to 6 h before sedation and from clear liquids for 2 h before sedation. Cow's milk and formula are considered to be solids, and breast milk is considered to be a clear liquid.

On the day of the imaging study, the history is reviewed and a focused clinical examination is performed by the radiology nurse or physician before sedation. The examination includes evaluation of the airway, cardiac status and neurological condition of the child. A history of previous sedation and any known airway risk factors should be established (Table 8.1). The child's fasting status should be confirmed. If they have eaten, they should not be sedated because of the risk of aspiration. In these circumstances, the study should either be delayed or rescheduled. In an emergency, sedation will need to be performed by anesthesia personnel.

Contraindications to sedation by radiology personnel include respiratory infection, compromised airway, a previous significant adverse reaction to sedatives, or significant underlying medical disease. The risk for sedation tends to correlate with the underlying health status.

Table 8.1 Causes of respiratory distress and airway compromise in children

Infection:	Bronchitis, croup, epiglottitis, pneumonia, retropharyngeal or tonsillar abscess
Intrinsic:	Asthma, reactive airways disease
Masses:	Cystic hygroma, lymphoma, adenopathy, abscess, rhabdomyosarcoma, hemangioma
Cardiac:	Congestive heart failure, vascular rings
Other:	Neuromuscular diseases, congenital anomalies, aspiration, sedation

The American Society of Anesthesiology (ASA) has classified patients into the following five groups:

- Class I – healthy patient;

- Class II – mild systemic disease, no functional limitation;

- Class III – severe systemic disease, definite functional limitation;

- Class IV – severe systemic disorder that is a constant threat to life;

- Class V – moribund patient with little chance of survival.

Conscious sedation by trained radiology personnel usually involves children in Classes I and II. Children in Classes III, IV and V are considered to be at high risk of complications.[7,8]

If the child's state of health is acceptable for conscious sedation, the planned sedation and risks are explained to the parent or caregiver and consent is obtained. If the child has significant risk factors such that the sedation procedure is beyond the ability of the radiology staff to perform safely, the examination or procedure should be rescheduled under the supervision of trained anesthesia personnel.

The radiology procedure area should be equipped with suction, oxygen, pediatric-sized oxygen delivery systems, and emergency pediatric medications. An emergency cart with pediatric intubation equipment should be readily available. Arrangements for backup assistance by pediatric-trained emergency personnel should be in place.

Medications

The foundation of a successful pediatric conscious sedation practice is the skilled, experienced use of a few carefully chosen sedative and analgesic agents. Most successful sedation procedures use only one or two drugs. The use of multiple drugs increases the risk of side-effects, and the sedation and respiratory depressive effects are often more than additive. Input and guidance from pediatric anesthesia personnel is invaluable when defining a few select drugs and developing medication dosage guidelines. The greater the communication between anesthesia and radiology personnel, the better the radiology sedation program will be.

The most commonly used drugs in radiology for pediatric conscious sedation include chloral hydrate, pentobarbital, midazolam and fentanyl (Table 8.2). *Propofol* is a relatively new and extremely effective sedative with valuable anesthetic properties. However, it is a potent respiratory depressant that necessitates continuous monitoring and dose titration and is best administered under the supervision of a nurse anesthetist or anesthesiologist.

Chloral hydrate is an effective oral sedative for infants and young toddlers.[9] It is a pure sedative, not an analgesic, and is not indicated to relieve pain in a painful

Table 8.2 Sedative agents

Agent	Class	Effect	Dose	Route	Onset	Duration
Chloral hydrate	Hypnotic	Sedative	25–100 mg/kg initial dose 25–50 mg infants 50–100 mg/kg older infants and toddlers Maximum *cumulative* dose: 100 mg/kg/day Maximum total dose: 2 g	PO (PR)	20–40 min	30–90 min
Pentobarbital sodium	Barbiturate	Sedative	2–3 mg/kg doses titrated 5–7 min until sedated Maximum *cumulative* dose: 7 mg/kg Maximum total dose: 200 mg	IV	5–10 min	40–60 min
Fentanyl citrate	Narcotic	Analgesic with sedative properties	0.5–1.0 μg/kg slowly Maximum *cumulative* dose: 2 μg/kg Maximum total dose: 2–20 μg/kg	IV	1–2 min	30–60 min for analgesia Sedation may be shorter
Midazolam	Benzodiazepine	Sedative, anxiolytic, amnestic	0.05–0.1 mg/kg Maximum *cumulative* dose: 0.2–0.3 mg/kg Maximum total dose: 5 mg	IV (PO)	1–5 min (IV)	20–30 min
			0.1–0.3 mg/kg 'one-off' (single) dose, Do not repeat	Intranasal	Variable	
Naloxone	NA	Narcotic antagonist	0.01–0.1 mg/kg (lower dose for infant) Repeat after 2–3 min Titrate to reversal Maximum dose: 2 mg	IV	1–2 min	Maximum 20–30 min
Flumazenil	NA	Benzodiazepine antagonist	Titrate to effect 0.01–0.02 mg/kg over 15–30 s Maximum initial dose: 0.2 mg Repeat doses of 0.005–0.01 mg/kg up to total *cumulative* dose of 1 mg	IV	1–3 min Peak effect in 6–10 min	30–60 min May need to repeat dose if resedation occurs

Table 8.2 *continued*

Agent	Class	Effect	Dose	Route	Onset	Duration

Atropine	Anticholinergic	Vagolytic	0.02 mg/kg IV
			Minimum initial
			  dose: 0.1 mg
			Maximum initial
			  dose:
			  0.5 mg (infants
			    and children)
			  1.0 mg (adolescents)
			Maximum total
			  dose 0.04 mg/kg:
			  for example,
			  1.0 mg (children)
			  2.0 mg (adolescents)
				IV	Peak effect
					  in 2–4 min	

NA, not applicable.

procedure. It is commonly used in children up to 12–18 months of age. In children older than this, the effect of chloral hydrate is more unpredictable. The dose of chloral hydrate is 25–100 mg/kg. Infants receive a lower initial dose of 25–50 mg/kg, while older infants and toddlers are initially given 50–100 mg/kg. The maximum cumulative dose is 100 mg/kg per day up to a maximum total dose of 2 g per day. There may be adverse effects such as nausea and vomiting, hyperactivity or respiratory depression in 7 per cent of children. On rare occasion, chloral hydrate has been associated with severe respiratory depression and should not be regarded as an absolutely safe drug with no adverse effects. Children receiving it fall within conscious sedation guidelines. Chloral hydrate is metabolized by the liver, and the dose should be reduced in children with underlying liver disease, as it may have a more profound and prolonged effect. Chloral hydrate is potentiated by benzodiazepines and barbiturates. If a chloral hydrate sedation fails at the maximum dose, the study should be rescheduled for another day, using a different sedative agent.

Due to the limited effect of chloral hydrate in children older than 18–24 months, intravenous sedation is commonly used for these children. The most commonly used drug for intravenous sedation in many radiology practices is the barbiturate *pentobarbital (Nembutal®)*, which is a short-acting barbiturate with a relatively wide safety margin. The usual starting dose of pentobarbital is 2–3 mg/kg IV. The dose can be slowly titrated over 10–30 min with a maximum cumulative dose of 7 mg/kg. The maximum total dose is 200 mg. Pentobarbital is metabolized by the liver, and the dose should be reduced in children with liver disease. The duration of action of the drug is 45–60 min. Prolonged sedation tends to be dose related. Recovery may be prolonged, lasting up to 2–3 h until the child fulfills the criteria for discharge. Uncommonly, a child may have to be admitted for overnight observation because of respiratory or central nervous system (CNS) depression.[10] Pentobarbital may cause a hyperexcitable phase at the beginning of sedation, and also as the child awakens from sedation. It may be difficult to restrain a large child or adolescent during this hyperexcitable phase, and alternative sedatives may need to be considered in this age group. Pentobarbital is a respiratory depressant and is potentiated when used in conjunction with benzodiazepines or narcotics, such as fentanyl. Its use is contraindicated in patients with a history of a previous idiosyncratic reaction or allergy to barbituates.

Fentanyl (Sublimaze®) is a narcotic that is rarely used alone in pediatric conscious sedation. It is most commonly used as an additive analgesic agent in conjunction with pentobarbital or midazolam. It is a potent respiratory depressant and should be given slowly. The usual dose of fentanyl is 0.5–1.0 μg/kg IV with incremental dosages of 0.5 μg/kg up to a maximum cumulative dose of 1–2 μg/kg. The ventilatory depressant action of fentanyl may last longer than the sedative effect. Children under 1 year of age are not given fentanyl because of their relatively immature respiratory system. When the narcotic fentanyl is used, the antagonist *naloxone (Narcan®)* should be immediately available. The dose of naloxone is 0.01–0.1 mg/kg. It may be repeated every 2–3 min and should be titrated to effect to reverse the respiratory depression. The maximum cumulative dose is 2.0 mg.

Midazolam (Versed®) is increasingly used for conscious sedation within radiology departments. Midazolam is a benzodiazepine that acts as a sedative and anxiolytic. It is not an analgesic, but it does have amnestic properties. It is a shorter-acting agent than pentobarbital and is therefore not as effective for sedating children for longer examinations, such as MRI. With the arrival of faster CT-scanning equipment and techniques, there is less need for prolonged patient immobility, and many studies can be completed in 5–10 min. Midazolam may be ideal for these studies because of its fast onset but short duration. Children who have been given this drug wake up relatively quickly with a short recovery time. The initial dose of midazolam is 0.05 mg/kg IV. It is a potent respiratory depressant and should be given slowly with increments of 0.05 mg up to a maximum cumulative dose of 0.2–0.3 mg/kg. Intranasal midazolam is occasionally used in some practices but can irritate the nasal mucosa. It is given as a 'one-off' (single) dose of 0.1–0.3 mg/kg. When midazolam is used, its reversal agent *flumazenil* should be immediately available. The dose of flumazenil is 0.01–0.02 mg/kg over 15–30 s. The maximum initial dose is 0.2 mg. Repeat doses of 0.005–0.01 mg/kg may be needed up to a total cumulative dose of 1 mg. The dose should be titrated to effect in order to overcome the respiratory depression produced by midazolam. The patient should be monitored closely for 2 h, as resedation may occur because midazolam has a longer duration of action than flumazenil.

Monitoring

The child must be monitored and vital signs documented throughout the sedation and recovery period. Monitoring includes continuous pulse oximetry for oxygen saturation and heart rate. Blood-pressure measurements are obtained both before the sedation and during recovery. They are not routinely checked during sedation if all other vital signs are stable, because cuff inflation may awaken a sleeping child. The respiratory rate is monitored visually.

Artificially low oxygen saturations may be the result of a poor fit of the pulse oximeter. Supplementary or 'blow-by' oxygen is routinely used and is helpful for maintaining adequate oxygen saturation levels. If the saturation dips down to 94 per cent or lower, it is appropriate to stop the study, readjust the child's head position, check the fit of the pulse oximeter, and increase oxygen delivery. Stimulation, although it has an adverse effect on the imaging study, may be needed to arouse the patient and improve oxygenation.

Uncommonly, the child may develop bradycardia during the course of sedation. If the heart rate falls below what is acceptable for the child's age (Table 8.3), atropine is given at a dose of 0.02 mg/kg IV with a maximum initial dose in an infant or child of 0.5 mg and in an adolescent of 1 mg. The minimum initial dose is 0.1 mg.

A trained staff member must stay with the child at all times and continuously assess the child throughout the radiologic examination and recovery period. The sedated child should be that individual's primary and only responsibility. The person responsible for the imaging or interventional procedure should not also be responsible for monitoring the sedated child.

Table 8.3 Normal vital signs by age

Age	Respiration rate (breaths/min)	Pulse rate (beats/min)
Newborn	30–60	100–160
1–6 weeks	30–60	100–160
6 months	25–40	90–140
1 year	20–40	90–130
3 years	20–30	80–120
6 years	12–25	70–110
10 years	12–20	60–90

Recovery

After the study, the child is monitored by trained members of the staff until the child is awake and alert or meets the baseline criteria. The Aldrete scoring system (Table 8.4) can be used as objective criteria to assess the child's status. A score of 8 out of 10 meets the discharge criteria. If the child does not meet the criteria for discharge, he or she may need to be admitted for observation.[11]

The child's parents or caregivers should be given oral and written discharge instructions, including a telephone number to call in case an emergency arises after discharge. The parents or caregivers should be informed that the sedated child may not have a complete return of protective reflexes for several hours, and

Table 8.4 Aldrete scoring system

	0	1	2
Activity	None	Limited	Normal
Respiration	Apneic	Shallow or dyspneic	Normal
Blood pressure	50% of baseline	50–80% of baseline	80% of baseline
Consciousness	Unresponsive	Sedate but arousable	Alert
Color	Cyanotic	Pale/dusky	Pink

may not be able to resume normal activities for the remainder of that day. Follow-up telephone calls by the nurse on the next day help to provide a more complete assessment of the sedation and any possible late complications. This call is also reassuring to the parents or caregivers.

Documentation

The entire presedation evaluation, sedation and monitoring, postsedation recovery and discharge condition and instructions must be documented in the child's medical record. A standard conscious sedation form is helpful for ensuring that all aspects of the sedation are documented. Such a standard form is also useful for quality assurance purposes. It is worthwhile keeping copies of the sedation record of each patient in the Radiology Department, since many children may undergo repeated imaging studies which require sedation.

Regular re-evaluation of the sedation guidelines and practice is needed for continual improvement and quality assurance. Review of problems, patient complaints, drugs and dosage schedules and adverse reactions is important for the success of the sedation practice.

Conclusion

Pediatric conscious sedation will continue to be needed in the radiology department in the foreseeable future. As long as pediatric conscious sedation is performed, radiology departments will need to develop and follow guidelines, document the sedation, and train and equip radiology personnel to care for the sedated child. This all serves to offer a high level of care for the sedated child, and to enable high-quality diagnostic studies to be performed.

References

1. Frush D, Bissett GS, Hall SC. Pediatric sedation in radiology: the practice of safe sleep. *American Journal of Roentgenology* 1996; **167**: 1381–7.

2. Maxwell LG, Yaste M. The myth of conscious sedation (editorial; comment). *Archives of Pediatric and Adolescent Medicine* 1996; **150**: 665–7.

3. Committee on Drugs. Guidelines for monitoring and management of pediatric patients during and after sedation for diagnostic and therapeutic procedures. *Pediatrics* 1992; **89**: 1110–15.

4. Joint Commission on Accreditation of Healthcare Organizations *1995 comprehensive accreditation manual for hospitals*. Oakbrook Terrace, IL: Joint Commission on Accreditation of Healthcare Organizations, 1998: 90–91.

5. Holzman RS, Cullen DJ, Eichhorn JH, Philip JH. Guidelines for sedation by nonanesthesiologists during diagnostic and therapeutic procedures. *Journal of Clinical Anesthesia* 1994; **6**: 265–76.

6. Cote CJ. Sedation for the pediatric patient. *Pediatric Clinics of North America* 1994; **41**: 31–58.

7. Dripps RD, Lamont A, Eckenhoff HE. The role of anesthesia in surgical mortality. *Journal of the American Medical Association* 1961; **178**: 261.

8. Miller RD, Ed. *Anesthesia*, 3rd edn. Edinburgh: Churchill Livingstone, 1990.

9. American Academy of Pediatrics Use of chloral hydrate for sedation in children. *Pediatrics* 1993; **92**: 471–3.

10. Egelhoff JC, Ball WS Jr, Koch BL, Parks TD. Safety and efficacy of sedation in children using a structured sedation program. *American Journal of Roentgenology* 1997; **168**: 1259–62.

11. Aldrete JA, Kroulik D. A postanesthetic recovery score. *Anesthesia and Analgesia* 1970; **49**: 924–34.

9 Contrast media extravasation

Richard H. Cohan

Introduction

Contrast media extravasation occurs occasionally in all radiology practices where radiographic contrast material is injected into the vascular system. The majority of extravasations involve small volumes of contrast media. Initial swelling usually diminishes promptly and, in most instances, resolves without any long-term sequelae. However, in rare instances severe tissue ulceration or necrosis result from even small volume ($\leq$ 10 mL) extravasations.[1,2] In one study, 31 patients suffering from major extravasation injuries (caused by a variety of agents) required an average of 3.5 operations per patient, prolonging the average hospital stay by 3 weeks.[3]

Incidence

Venography
The frequency of contrast media extravasations varies to some extent with the type of study being performed. They are most frequent during ascending lower extremity venography, where injections are performed on edematous extremities, often while tourniquets are applied. Venous access can be tenuous. In Gothlin's study, extravasation (usually of small volumes) developed in 28 of 36 patients (78 per cent) who received contrast material through a needle puncturing the dorsal vein of the large toe.[4] When a catheter was used for injection, extravasation occurred in only 8 of 176 patients (4.5 per cent).[4]

Computed tomography
Although the number of contrast media extravasations during CT has increased substantially over the past few years as dynamic bolus techniques with automated injectors have become widely used, the overall incidence of extravascular injection remains considerably lower than that observed with venography. Extravasation has been estimated to occur during 0.04 to 0.4 per cent of CT examinations.[5-8]

There is a significant potential for large-volume extravasation during dynamic bolus CT. The contrast injection is not usually completed before image acquisition has commenced, and close inspection of the intravenous access site is not feasible for most of the injection period. Of 39 recently published cases of contrast media extravasations during CT, 16 (41 per cent) involved volumes of 50 mL or more.[5-7]

Urography

Extravasation during urography has also been described, although with less frequency, and there are only two recent reports in the literature.[1,9] While many cases are not publicized, it is probable that the relatively easy venous access in most patients and the ability to monitor patients closely throughout contrast media injection is responsible for the dearth of significant extravasations.

Mechanism

A considerable number of adults with indwelling intravenous lines develop fluid extravasations,[10] many of which apparently develop as a result of a phlebitis induced by the presence of the venous catheter.[11] The cannulated vein eventually becomes narrowed due to inflammation or spasm. Increased pressure is required for intravenous infusion. Fluid then leaks back through the single hole created by the correctly positioned line. In general, the intravenous line must be in place for about 20 h before this type of phlebitis can develop.[11]

It is presumed that most contrast media extravasations result either from the creation of two holes in a vein (double-wall puncture or multiple consecutive punctures) or from actual placement of the needle or catheter tip outside a vein. Extravasation of contrast media through a single defect in an inflamed vein would only be expected if a pre-existing intravenous line is employed for injection.

Risk factors

Some patients are more likely to develop extravasation. Patients at the extremes of age or who are unconscious are less likely to complain of injection-site pain.[10] Extravasation is more likely to occur in patients who are injected through small peripheral veins, in cases where tourniquets are not released, and in patients with indwelling intravenous lines.[3] In addition to being located in phlebitic veins, pre-existing intravenous lines may become dislodged while the patient is being transferred to the radiology department.[3] While backflow of blood should be obtained through tubing connected to any indwelling line prior to the injection of contrast material, its presence does not guarantee adequate positioning.[10] Tapes and bandages may cover the skin directly over an intravenous access site, making visual and even tactile inspection of the area during injection impossible.

Multiple attempts to establish intravenous access through the same vein can also be a problem.[3] Contrast material that is properly instilled through a peripheral vein may leak out of a defect that has just been created more centrally. It is therefore preferable to proceed more centrally or to a site that has different venous drainage when initial punctures that traverse one or both walls of a vein cannot be used.

Extravasation is more likely to occur during an injection through a metal needle than during one through a plastic cannula.[3] This probably reflects an intrinsic technical advantage of the latter over the former.[4] It is also possible that metal needles (e.g. 'butterflies') are more likely to be used in patients whose intravenous access sites are more tenuous (i.e. smaller veins).

Incidence of serious injuries

Venography

The frequency of significant skin or subcutaneous tissue damage resulting from contrast media extravasation has only been determined for ascending lower extremity venography. Berge et al.[12] and Thomas[13] noted that skin necrosis developed after ascending lower extremity venography performed with non-dilute (60 per cent by weight) ionic contrast media in 0.4 and 0.5 per cent of their patients, respectively. If clinically insignificant extravasation occurs with an incidence comparable to that observed by Gothlin,[4] it can be estimated that between one in 10 and one in 200 extravascular injections of standard concentrations of ionic agents can be expected to result in a severe injury during venography. These data are consistent with observations of extravasation of chemotherapeutic agents. In a large sample of 119 patients who had extravasations while receiving chemotherapy, 11 per cent had injuries that were severe enough to require operative intervention.[14]

Computed tomography

None of the previously cited 39 extravasations of contrast media during CT resulted in skin ulceration or subcutaneous tissue necrosis.[5-7] This is probably due to the fact that 36 of 39 patients received nonionic agents, which are better tolerated. In anecdotal case reports of severe damage resulting from injection of contrast media for CT,[10,15-18] in three cases the injury was caused by nonionic agents.[16-18]

Mechanisms of severe injury

Although it is generally believed that the hyperosmolality of contrast media is primarily responsible for its extravascular toxicity,[10] additional factors are probably involved. Kim et al.[19] found that 2100, 1500 and 60 mOsm/kg concentrations of sodium meglumine ioxithalamate (a conventional ionic agent) were all more toxic to cutaneous tissues than equiosmolar injections of sodium chloride in rats. This additional adverse effect may be due to any of a number of factors, including molecular structure (direct cytotoxicity), ionicity or viscosity. When large volumes are extravasated, simple mechanical compression may also be a factor.[3] In addition, once skin ulceration and necrosis occur, the extravasation site may become super-infected.[3]

Risk factors for severe injuries

Patients who have had previous radiation therapy to an injection site, patients with arterial insufficiency (e.g. atherosclerosis. diabetes mellitus, or connective tissue diseases such as Raynaud's syndrome), and patients with central or peripheral venous thrombosis are all at increased risk of a severe complication from an extravascular injection of contrast media.[3] In Gothlin and Hallbrook's series, [20] all four patients who developed skin necrosis after extravasation during venography had reduced lower extremity circulation.

Significant morbidity from an extravasation is more likely to result when injections are performed into the dorsum of the hand, foot or ankle, because of the small amount of subcutaneous tissue and the close proximity of tendons, blood vessels and nerves.[2,3] For this reason, the antecubital fossae and forearms should be checked first when searching for a suitable location for venapuncture.

It is also generally acknowledged that larger volumes of extravasated contrast medium are more likely to cause tissue damage.

Low-osmolality contrast media

Some studies have shown that low-osmolality contrast media are better tolerated than conventional ionic contrast media when extravasated in animals.[19,21] Extravascular nonionic contrast media are also considered to be extremely safe in humans. All of five intermediate or large-volume (18–150 mL) extravasations of nonionic contrast media during dynamic CT reported by Cohan et al. resolved uneventfully.[5] More recently, 28 nonionic contrast media extravasations observed by Sistrom et al.,[7] and 37 nonionic contrast agent extravasations reported by Cohan et al. during dynamic CT,[8] did not cause lasting damage to the skin or subcutaneous tissues.

To date, there have been only three reports of injuries produced by extravasated nonionic contrast media. One of these involved the development of skin ulceration after extravasation of 150 mL from an upper extremity injection site.[16] The extravasation occurred while an automatic blood-pressure cuff was left inflated during the injection. In the second case, a 'compartment syndrome' resulted from injection of over 100 mL of a nonionic agent into a patient's forearm.[17] The third case involved extravasation of 60 mL of ioversol 320 mg/mL into the dorsum of the hand during a CT examination, which produced swelling and blistering. A 'compartment syndrome' developed, necessitating an emergency fasciotomy.[18]

Magnetic resonance imaging (MRI) agents

Animal studies have demonstrated that gadopentetate dimeglumine, the most widely used MRI contrast agent, is capable of producing skin ulceration and necrosis, although it appears to be somewhat better tolerated than conventional ionic radiographic contrast media.[22,23] Since small volumes of MRI agents are usually injected, serious injuries resulting from extravascular injections of ionic, high-osmolality gadopentetate dimeglumine should be much less frequently encountered than those seen after extravasation of iodinated radiographic contrast media. Interestingly, gadoteridol – a nonionic MRI agent – was found to be no more toxic than normal saline when injected subcutaneously in rats.[23]

Presentation

Once extravasation occurs, nearly all patients have the same signs and symptoms.[24] They often complain of stinging or burning pain, and the affected site may become erythematous, swollen and tender.[24] Laboratory studies[25] and clinical observations[3] have suggested that there is an initial tendency to underestimate the severity of an extravasation injury, since the most severe manifestations may not be apparent for 48 to 72 h.

Rarely, patients may develop acute local pain or erythema during or immediately after injection of a substance through a correctly positioned venous catheter, possibly due to irritation of the vascular endothelium.[26] This was observed primarily during the era of high-osmolality ionic contrast agents. The phlebitis can usually be distinguished from an extravasation because the intravenous line is functioning properly and there is no soft tissue swelling. The local pain often subsides quickly. Delayed injection-site pain, beginning between 30 min and 2 days after contrast media injection, has also been observed.[27] Delayed local pain may last for several days, but essentially it always resolves after about 1 month.

Treatment

While there have been many studies of therapy of extravasation injuries produced by chemotherapeutic agents, data on the treatment of contrast media extravasations have been sparse. Currently, there is no widely accepted treatment regimen.

Medical therapy

The few animal studies involving non-surgical treatment of contrast media extravasation sites have yielded conflicting results. This is not entirely surprising, given the wide variation in methodology employed. It must also be emphasized that the studies summarized below were all performed in rodents, whose skin differs markedly from that of humans.

Elevation

Elevation of the affected extremity is thought to reduce swelling by decreasing hydrostatic pressure in the capillaries. Soft-tissue swelling at the site of extravasation may therefore be reduced and resorption promoted. Despite these clinical effects, the efficacy of extremity elevation is uncertain.

Topical heat or cold

Elam *et al.* reported that skin ulcers in mice, which developed after diatrizoate (conventional ionic contrast medium) extravasation, could be reduced in size by exposing the injection site to a condom filled with cold water (17°C) for 20 min.[28] Conversely, Park *et al.* observed that the severity of injury in rats receiving subcutaneous injections of ioxithalamate (conventional ionic contrast medium) was not affected by the immediate application of cold water (7–12°C) for 10 min.[29] In neither Elam's nor Park's experiments was topical heat (43–44°C and 34–40°C, respectively) of any benefit.

Local dilution

The efficacy of local dilution of the extravasated contrast material has been evaluated and the results are again conflicting. In two studies, injection of additional saline modestly but significantly reduced the severity of damage caused by deep dermal injections of diatrizoate in rats.[29,30] However, in another similar study, no histologic advantage to diluting extravasated contrast medium was observed.[24] Even if local dilution is helpful in humans, the volumes used in animal studies are so large that such treatment may often not be practicable. For example, in the study by Park *et al.*, the volume of diluent evaluated was equal to 50 per cent of the volume of contrast medium extravasated (0.3 mL vs. 0.6 mL).[29] If these results are translated into clinically relevant volumes, a 50-mL contrast medium extravasation site would have to be injected with 25 mL of saline or water in order to maximize the benefit of local dilution. A radiologist might be reluctant to administer such a significant amount of additional fluid because of concern about exacerbating any pressure effects on the skin or other structures.

Local injections of antidotes

Local injections of potential antidotes to reduce the severity of injuries produced by chemotherapeutic agents have also given mixed results. Topical instillation of hyaluronidase has been reported to reduce the size of ulcers produced by contrast media extravasations in mice,[25] but significantly increased the inflammatory reaction at extravasation sites in rats.[24] Hyaluronidase is an enzyme that breaks down the connective tissue mycopolysaccharide, hyaluronic acid. Large volumes and high concentrations of hyaluronidase have usually been necessary for effectiveness.[24,25] Local injection of corticosteroids has been reported to have no effect on contrast medium-induced extravasation injuries in animal studies.[29, 30]

Surgery

Surgical drainage of an extravasation site is nearly always effective, and has been recommended by some authorities for any contrast medium extravasation in excess of 20 mL.[15] Others have recently shown that liposuction or copious saline irrigation reduce the likelihood of significant morbidity from a contrast medium extravasation.[2] Liposuction is performed through a single incision adjacent to the area of extravasation. Saline irrigation has been performed via four small local incisions through each of which a blunt-ended needle is inserted; 500 mL of fluid are then used to wash out the affected area.[2]

Early detection of extravasation

Recent work has suggested that microwave radiometry may be used to detect small changes in skin temperature resulting from extravasation of minimal amounts of contrast medium.[31] Such an extravasation 'detector' has been successfully linked to automated injectors in animal studies.[31] The 'detector' works by triggering an alarm and abruptly terminating a contrast injection once a few milliliters of contrast medium appear adjacent to rather than within a vein. Other studies have demonstrated that pressure tracings in malfunctioning intravenous lines differ from those in functioning lines.[32] More recently, an extravasation detector linked to a mechanical injector has become commercially available.

Suggested management of contrast media extravasations

It is not clear whether any local treatment except surgery is effective for contrast media extravasation injuries. Therefore it is best to prevent the injury from occurring in the first place. Patients at increased risk of extravasation and severe injury from extravasation (Table 9.1) should be injected carefully. Situations that are more likely to result in extravasation (Table 9.1) should be avoided if at all possible. If contrast medium is required in high-risk settings, the use of low-osmolality contrast material (particularly nonionic agents) is recommended.

Table 9.1 Risk factors for extravasation and extravasation injuries

---

Abnormal circulation in limb to be injected
  Atherosclerotic peripheral vascular disease
  Connective tissue disease
  Diabetic vascular disease
  Previous radiation
  Tourniquets
  Venous thrombosis

Noncommunicative patients
  Demented
  Elderly
  Infants and children
  Unconscious

Problems at the site to be injected
  Injections through needles (rather than catheters)
  Injections on dorsum of hand, foot or ankle
  Multiple punctures of the same vein
  Use of indwelling intravenous lines (particularly when in place for more than 20 h)

Note: consider using nonionic contrast media or dilute ionic media in the above situations, particularly if intravenous access is difficult.

We recommend that all radiologists who use radiographic contrast material intravascularly have a policy for dealing with extravasation injuries when they occur (Table 9.2). This policy should be developed in conjunction with those physicians who would have to treat the patient with a major extravasation injury. The policy should include provision for close monitoring of patients after any extravasation injury.

If an extravasation occurs at our institution, the affected extremity is elevated above the heart in such a way that the circulation to and from that extremity is not compromised. Ice packs are applied for 15–60 min. These applications can be repeated two or three times a day if necessary.

Patients are then monitored in the radiology department for approximately 2–4 h. The extravasation site is inspected periodically for any increase in swelling or pain, altered tissue sensation or perfusion, and skin ulceration or blistering. The plastic surgery service is consulted immediately if a patient develops these signs or symptoms. In addition, plastic surgery consultation is requested for any extravasated volume estimated to exceed 30 mL of conventional ionic contrast medium or 100 mL of nonionic contrast medium. These values are admittedly arbitrary. If the patient's symptoms are mild and do not worsen over time, and if the extravasated volumes are low, the patient can be discharged. The patient is given a telephone number to call if his or her status changes. A physician or nurse also routinely contacts the patient at least once every 24 h until the patient's signs and symptoms have disappeared completely. During these conversations, the

Table 9.2   Policy for treatment of extravasation injuries

Immediate treatment
    Elevation of affected extremity (above heart)
    Ice packs (15–60 min applications)
    Call referring physician (for any extravasation exceeding 5 mL)
    Observation for 2–4 h (if volume exceeds 5 mL)
    Local hyaluronidase injections (controversial)

Indications for plastic surgery consultation
    Extravasated volume exceeds 30 mL conventional ionic or 100 mL nonionic contrast
       material
    Patient develops any of the following: skin blistering or ulceration; altered tissue
       perfusion, sensation or temperature; increasing or persistent pain

Daily telephone calls by nurse or radiologist until manifestations resolve.
    Assess:
        1 residual pain;
        2 blistering or ulceration;
        3 redness or other skin color change;
        4 altered consistency, temperature or sensation.

Documentation
    Contrast extravasation report form
    Progress note in clinical record

---

patient is asked whether the pain is increasing and whether there is any blistering, ulceration, color, temperature or consistency change at the injured area. If the patient answers affirmatively to any of these questions, he or she is asked to return to the hospital for further evaluation. Complete documentation of this process is also required. A contrast extravasation report form is completed by the physician, nurse or technician who witnesses the extravasation, and the incident is also summarized in the clinical record. The radiologist is also expected to notify the referring physician when the volume of extravasated contrast material is in excess of 5 mL.

Summary

Significant injuries resulting from extravascular injections of contrast media are fortunately very rare. However, all radiologists must be prepared to follow and treat patients when these complications occur. In addition, attempts should be made to minimize the likelihood of extravasation and severe injuries from extravasation by taking extra care when injecting patients who are identified as being at increased risk. It is extremely helpful to have a policy in place for dealing with contrast media extravasation.

References

1. Ayre-Smith G. Tissue necrosis following extravasation of contrast media. *Journal of the Canadian Association of Radiologists* 1982; **33**: 104.

2. Gault DT. Extravasation injuries. *British Journal of Plastic Surgery* 1993; **46**: 91–6.

3. Upton J, Mulliken JB, Murray JE. Major intravenous extravasation during peripheral phlebography. *American Journal of Surgery* 1979; **137**: 497–506.

4. Gothlin J. The comparative frequency of extravasal injection at phlebography with steel and plastic cannula. *Clinical Radiology* 1972; **23**: 183–4.

5. Cohan RH, Dunnick NR, Leder RA, Baker ME. Extravasation of nonionic radiologic contrast media: efficiency of conservative treatment. *Radiology* 1990; **174**: 65–7.

6. Miles SG, Rasmussen JF, Litwiller T. Safe use of an intravenous power injector for CT: experience and protocol. *Radiology* 1990; **176**: 69–70.

7. Sistrom CL, Gay SB, Peffley L. Extravasation of iopamidol and iohexol during contrast-enhanced CT: report of 28 cases. *Radiology* 1991; **180**: 707–10.

8. Cohan RH, Bullard MA, Ellis JH, Jan SH, Francis IR, Garner WL, Dunnick NR. Local reactions after injection of iodinated contrast material: detection, management, outcome. *Academic Radiology* 1997; **4**: 711–18.

9. Leung PC, Cheng CY. Extensive local necrosis following the intravenous use of X-ray contrast medium in the upper extremity. *British Journal of Radiology* 1980; **53**: 361–4.

10. Burd DAR, Santis G, Milward TM. Severe extravasation injury: an avoidable iatrogenic disaster. *British Medical Journal* 1985; **290**: 1579–80.

11. Lewis GBH, Hector JF. Radiological examination of failure of intravenous infusions. *British Journal of Surgery* 1991; **78**: 500–501.

12. Berge T, Bergovist D, Efsing HO, Hallbrook T. Local complications of ascending phlebography. *Clinical Radiology* 1978; **29**: 691–6.

13. Thomas ML. Gangrene following peripheral phlebography of the legs. *British Journal of Radiology* 1970; **43**: 528–30.

14. Larson DL. What is the appropriate management of tissue extravasation by antitumor agents? *Plastic and Reconstructive Surgery* 1985; **75**: 397.

15. Loth TS, Jones DEC. Extravasations of radiographic contrast material in the upper extremity. *Journal of Hand Surgery: American volume* 1988; **13**: 395–8.

16. Pond GD, Dorr RT, McAleese KA. Skin ulceration from extravasation of low-osmolality contrast medium: a complication of automation. *American Journal of Roentgenology* 1992; **158**: 915–16.

17. Memolo M, Dyer R, Zagoria RJ. Extravasation injury with nonionic contrast material. *American Journal of Roentgenology* 1993; **160**: 203.

18. Young RA. Injury due to extravasation of nonionic contrast material (letter). *American Journal of Roentgenology* 1994; **162**: 1499.

19. Kim SH, Park JH, Kim YI, Kim CW, Han MC. Experimental tissue damage after subcutaneous injection of water-soluble contrast media. *Investigative Radiology* 1990; **25**: 678–85.

20. Gothlin J, Hallbrook T. Skin necrosis following extravasal injection of contrast medium at phlebography. *Der Radiologe* 1971; **1**: 161–5.

21. Cohan RH, Leder RA, Bolick D et al. Extravascular extravasation of radiographic contrast media. Effects of conventional and low-osmolar agents in the rat thigh. *Investigative Radiology* 1990; **25**: 504–10.

22. McAlister WH, McAlister VI, Kissane JM. The effect of Gd-dimeglumine on subcutaneous tissues: a study with rats. *American Journal of Neuroradiology* 1990; **11**: 325–7.

23. Cohan RH, Leder RA, Herzberg AJ et al. Extravascular toxicity of two magnetic resonance contrast agents: preliminary experience in the rat. *Investigative Radiology* 1991; **26**: 224–6.

24. Heckler FR. Current thoughts on extravasation injuries. *Clinics in Plastic Surgery* 1989; **16**: 557–63.

25. McCallister WH, Palmer K. The histologic effects of four commonly used media for excretory urography and an attempt to modify the responses. *Radiology* 1971; **99**: 511–16.

26. Shehadi WH. Adverse reactions to intravascularly administered contrast media: a comprehensive study based on a prospective survey. *Radiology* 1975; **124**: 145–52.

27. Yoshikawa H. Late adverse reactions to nonionic contrast media. *Radiology* 1992; **183**: 737–40.

28. Elam EA, Dorr RT, Lagel KE, Pond GD. Cutaneous ulceration due to contrast extravasation: experimental assessment of injury and potential antidotes. *Investigative Radiology* 1991; **26**: 13–16.

29. Park KS, Kim SH, Park JH, Han MC, Kim DY, Kim SJ. Methods for mitigating soft-tissue injury after subcutaneous injection of water-soluble contrast media. *Investigative Radiology* 1993; **28**: 332–4.

30. Cohan RH, Leder RA, Herzberg AJ, Hedlund LW, Beam CA, Dunnick NR. Treatment of injuries induced by extravasation of radiologic contrast media. Paper presented at the 38th Annual Meeting of the Association of Radiologists, Minneapolis, MN, April 1990.

31. Shaeffer J, Sigfred SV, Sevcik MA, Grabowy RS, Gemmell LA, Hirschmann AD. Early detection of radiographic contrast medium: work in progress. *Radiology* 1992; **184**: 141–4.

32. Phelps SJ, Tolley EA. Infusion technology for predicting and detecting infiltration of peripheral intravenous catheter sites in infants. *Clinical Pharmacy* 1993; **12**: 216–21.

10 Contrast nephrotoxicity

Henrik S. Thomsen

Contrast-medium nephropathy is defined as acute renal impairment that occurs after exposure to contrast media and for which other causes have been eliminated.[1,2] It is a diagnosis of exclusion. On CT it may be diagnosed by the finding of persistent cortical and corticomedullary attenuation differences 24 h after the administration of the contrast agent (Fig. 10.1). On conventional radiographs a 'white' kidney is present bilaterally. However, a persistent bilateral nephrogram may also be seen in bilateral obstruction and in hypotension. If the parenchymal accumulation is unilateral, it is usually due to obstruction (e.g. renal colic), and accumulation of contrast material will also occur in the renal pelvis. Other

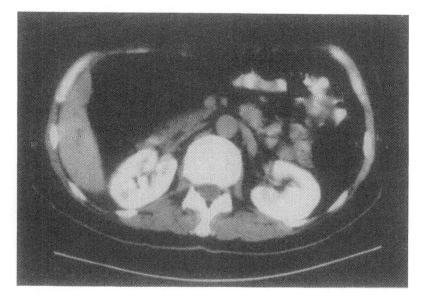

Figure 10.1 Contrast-induced nephrotoxicity: persistent nephrogram. CT scan performed 24 h after arterial administration of a contrast medium in a patient with diabetic nephropathy. There is bilateral parenchymal accumulation, especially in the cortex, but no contrast evident in the renal pelvis.

processes (vascular impairment or infection) should be considered in the differential diagnosis.

How important is contrast nephrotoxicity?

Contrast-induced nephropathy is a major problem for the affected patient, but is an infrequent complication of contrast-material use, affecting less than 1 per cent of low-risk patients. In high-risk groups (< 5 per cent of examined patients), it may be seen in 5–90 per cent of patients, depending on the subgroup.[1] In patients with diabetic nephropathy the risk is very high. Conversely, in patients with obstructive nephropathy the risk is much lower. When contrast nephrotoxicity is detected (e.g. as an increase in serum creatinine levels of > 100 µmol/L [1.1 mg/dL]) the clinician faces a major question. Is it a permanent or temporary decrease in renal function? Acute serum creatinine elevation of ⩾ 100 µmol/L (1.1 mg/dL) following contrast administration commonly leads to additional laboratory testing, postponement of further radiographic contrast exposure or surgical interventions, and often prolongation of hospitalization. For a patient with poor renal function (glomerular filtration rate (GFR) of 3–9 mL/min), loss of 1–3 mL/min in renal function may necessitate dialysis, which is often permanent. For the patient with renal function above 100 mL/min GFR, a temporary loss of 1–3 mL/min will not be detected. For patients on peritoneal dialysis, loss of 1–3 mL/min in residual function of their own kidneys may necessitate hemodialysis. Hemodialysis is extremely expensive and necessitates the patient being connected to the machine for hours, two or three times a week.

Why is the kidney at risk?

There are several reasons for renal susceptibility to toxic challenge.

1 The kidneys represent 0.4 per cent of body mass and receive 20–25 per cent of resting cardiac output per minute, so all blood-borne solutes are delivered rapidly to the renal parenchyma.

2 High rates of renal oxygen consumption produce sensitivity to agents that impair cellular uptake or utilization of oxygen.

3 Some solutes are reabsorbed from the nephron's luminal fluid, further increasing the concentration in parenchymal cells.

4 Other solutes are secreted into the nephron's luminal fluid, thereby increasing the concentration near the luminal cell membranes.

5 The solute concentration is further increased by the action of antidiuretic hormone.

6 Certain compounds taken up by renal cells are retained for long periods of time, so that both solute concentrations and duration of toxic exposure are increased.

7 Patients with a reduced nephron population excrete all solutes through fewer nephrons, thereby increasing the dose per nephron.

8 Volume depletion, or obstruction to flow of urine, may lead to greater reabsorption of a solute or to prolonged exposure of susceptible tissue to a toxic solute.

History

In the 1970s and 1980s, contrast studies were implicated as the cause of 12 per cent of cases of hospital-acquired renal insufficiency.[3] Whether the use of lower osmolality, nonionic contrast media and increased awareness of the risk of contrast nephrotoxicity will be found to have reduced the frequency in the 1990s is unknown. In the 1950s it was widely believed that administration of contrast media was relatively contraindicated in cases of renal impairment because it was unlikely that useful information would be obtained with intravenous urography, and because use of the contrast media would probably cause further deterioration in renal function. In the early 1960s, studies showed that when radiologists used a high dose of contrast medium in patients with renal failure, they could obtain a nephrogram and pyelogram that were sufficiently satisfactory to provide information that might alter management. More recently, the safety of contrast media in renal failure has become less certain.

Risk factors

Factors that increase the risk of contrast-medium nephropathy are being identified more specifically.[4-6] Pre-existing renal impairment (serum creatinine >132 μmol/L [1.5 mg/dL]) is the most significant risk factor, followed by albuminuria (> 2+), hypertension, age > 60 years, dehydration, uric acid (> 8.0 mg/dL) and multiple closely spaced doses of iodinated contrast material. Other risk factors include severe congestive heart failure, reduced effective arterial volume (as occurs in nephrosis and cirrhosis), multiple myeloma, and administration of a single high dose of contrast agent. Concomitant use of drugs that impair renal responses, such as angiotensin-converting-enzyme inhibitors (ACEI), antibiotics such as gentamicin, and non-steroidal anti-inflammatory drugs (NSAIDs) also increase the risk. Because many patients have more than one risk factor, it is not possible to determine the independent contribution of each factor to the development of renal failure. It is generally accepted that the coexistence of several of the factors increases the risk of contrast-induced nephropathy considerably. For example, a patient with diabetic nephropathy generally has at least three risk factors, namely reduced renal function, albuminuria and hypertension.

Incidence

The true incidence of contrast-induced nephropathy cannot be established with certainty because data reported in different studies vary depending on the population studied and the definition of acute renal dysfunction adopted in the study. Furthermore, systematic monitoring of renal function after contrast administration is not performed routinely. If it is monitored, it is very rarely followed for 5 consecutive days.

Clinically, glomerular filtration rate is usually assessed indirectly by measuring the serum creatinine concentration or by measuring creatinine clearance. This operational definition may greatly underestimate toxic results that are not severe enough to affect these insensitive markers of renal function. Serum creatinine concentration – the measure most often used as an indicator of renal dysfunction – depends on muscle mass and may not become elevated above the normal range until the glomerular filtration rate falls to 50 per cent of normal, because of its non-linear relationship to glomerular filtration rate. Serum creatinine as a measure of renal function cannot reveal toxic insults that lower functional reserve capacity. An unchanged serum creatinine concentration after administration of a contrast medium does not exclude the presence of long-term effects. Moreover, endogenous serum creatinine clearance as a measure of GFR is inaccurate, especially when the level of renal function is low, because a compensatory increase in tubular secretion negates the validity of serum creatinine as a glomerular filtration marker.[7] Retrospective studies usually underestimate the true incidence of contrast nephropathy, and prospective studies yield different estimates of the incidence of contrast nephropathy, apparently because of differences in patient selection, state of hydration, rate and site of administration, dose of contrast medium, and variable definitions of acute renal failure. The definitions used in various studies and reports have included increases in serum creatinine concentration of 26 μmol/L,[8,9] 44 μmol/L,[10,11] 50 μmol/L,[12] 88 μmol/L,[13–15] and 176 μmol/L,[16,17] or a 50 per cent increase[18,19] in the baseline creatinine concentration from 1 to 5 days after patients' exposure to contrast media.[18,19]

When contrast nephrotoxicity occurs, the serum creatinine level usually begins to increase within the first 24 to 48 h and peaks from 96 to 120 h after administration of the contrast media. Although it commonly returns to baseline within 7 to 10 days, renal failure requiring short-term or even chronic dialysis is not an infrequent outcome in high-risk groups, e.g. patients with diabetic nephropathy and poor renal function.

Pathophysiology

Contrast media may have adverse effects on different parts of the kidney. When contrast material reaches the glomerulus, almost all of it is filtered through the glomerular basement membrane. During passage through the glomerular basement membrane, contrast media may affect the glomerular filter, as is illustrated by dramatically increased albuminuria during the first few hours after injection of some types of contrast media. Whether increased albuminuria following contrast-medium administration has any association with the occurrence of contrast-medium nephropathy is still unknown. When descending within the nephron, contrast media are concentrated. Starting with a concentration of a few mg/mL of iodine in the proximal tubules, the concentration may reach several hundred mg/mL of iodine (0.1–0.5 M) in the collecting tubules. Due to the osmotic properties of contrast media, low-osmolar contrast media will be concentrated more than twice as much as high-osmolar contrast media. These very high molar concentrations, which are higher still in the dehydrated patient, mean that contrast media must have low inherent chemotoxicity, especially the nonionic low-osmolality and the nonionic iso-osmolal contrast media. Because contrast agents are not reabsorbed by the nephron, the increase in fluid reabsorption during dehydration will increase the intratubular concentration of the contrast medium along the proximal tubule.

Over the years many mechanisms have been proposed to explain contrast-medium-induced nephropathy.[1] Currently all of the evidence points towards the tubular cells as the area where injury occurs. Whether it is an indirect effect (through the vascular bed) or a direct one (chemotoxicity) has yet to be elucidated. The indirect mechanism is probably mediated through vasoconstrictors such as adenosine or endothelin, as they both decrease renal blood flow and glomerular filtration pressure, resulting in a decrease in glomerular filtration rate, often manifested as an increase in serum creatinine levels. Vasoconstriction may lead to general or regional hypoxia.

Prevention

Several measures have been recommended to prevent contrast-medium-induced nephropathy, including hydration with 0.9 per cent NaCl or 0.45 per cent NaCl, infusion of mannitol, infusion of atrial natriuretic factor (ANF), administration of loop diuretics, calcium antagonists, theophylline, dopamine, use of low-osmolality, nonionic contrast media (LOCM) instead of high-osmolality ionic contrast media (HOCM), hemodialysis immediately after contrast administration, limiting the volume of contrast medium used, and prolonging the interval between doses of contrast. Extracellular volume expansion has repeatedly been shown to be effective and is the most widely recommended preventive measure.[20] Patients with pre-existing renal failure, independent of cause, should be well hydrated before and after administration of contrast medium,[20] the only exception to this being the patient with congestive heart failure. For patients who are unable to drink or eat prior to an interventional or surgical procedure, adequate hydration may be maintained through intravenous administration of 100 mL/h of normal or half-normal saline starting 4 h before contrast-medium administration and continuing for 24 h after the procedure. Patients who can and may drink should have at least the same volume, namely 500 mL of water or soft drinks before the procedure and 2500 mL during the following 24 h. In warm climates, more fluid should be given. These amounts should cover normal body losses (perspiration, respiration) and secure a diuresis of at least 1 mL/min. Furthermore, nonionic low-osmolar contrast media should always be used, since the incidence of acute nephrotoxicity in high-risk patients is significantly lower with nonionic contrast media compared to conventional, high-osmolality ionic contrast media.[21,22] The interval between two examinations in which contrast media are administered should be at least 48 h. Concomitant use of nephrotoxic drugs (e.g. gentamicin, NSAIDs) should be avoided.

MRI contrast media

To date there is no evidence that the current gadolinium-containing contrast media for magnetic resonance imaging (MRI) are more nephrotoxic than the iodinated contrast media in equimolar doses.[23] The customary molar dose of MRI contrast media is about one-tenth that of conventional iodinated contrast media, which is apparently very advantageous. When standard iodinated contrast media are used in the same very low molar doses (e.g. for determination of glomerular filtration rate, 3–7 gI) as are used with gadolinium-containing agents for MRI (0.1 mmol/kg), no nephrotoxic effects are observed.[24,25] In a retrospective study of 64 patients exposed to both iodinated contrast medium (50–60 gI) and MRI contrast medium (0.2–0.4 mmol/kg) on separate occasions, only after the administration of the iodinated contrast medium was an increase in serum creatinine levels observed, but equimolar doses of these two types of contrast agents were not used.[26] When MRI contrast medium is excreted slowly in patients with poor renal function (GFR < 10 mL/min), it has no detectable adverse effects.[27] MRI contrast agents can be easily removed by routine hemodialysis.[27] If it is possible to choose between CT and MRI for a patient at high risk for contrast nephrotoxicity, MRI is preferred.

References

1. Thomsen HS, Golman K, Hemmingsen L, Larsen S, Skaarup P, Svendsen O. Contrast medium-induced nephropathy: animal experiments. *Frontiers in European Radiology* 1993; **9**: 83–108.

2. Thomsen HS. Contrast nephropathy. *Current Opinion in Radiology* 1990; **2**: 793–802.

3. Hou SH, Bushinsky DA, Wish JB, Cohan JJ, Harrington JT. Hospital–acquired renal insufficiency: a prospective study. *American Journal of Medicine* 1983; **74**: 243–8.

4. Berns AS. Nephrotoxicity of contrast media. *Kidney International* 1989; **36**: 730–40.

5. Cronin RE. Renal failure following radiologic procedures. *American Journal of the Medical Sciences* 1989; **298**: 342–56.

6. Porter GA. Contrast-associated nephropathy. *American Journal of Cardiology* 1989; **64**: 22E–26E.

7. Blaufox MD, Aurell M, Bubeck B *et al.* Renal clearance: Report of the Radionuclides in Nephrourology Committee. *Journal of Nuclear Medicine* 1996; **37**: 1883–1890.

8. Older RA, Miller JP, Jackson DC, Johnsrude IS, Thompson WM. Angiographically-induced renal failure and its radiographic detection. *American Journal of Roentgenology* 1976; **126**: 1039–45.

9. Cochran ST, Wong WS, Roe DJ. Predicting angiography-induced acute renal function impairment. Clinical risk model. *American Journal of Roentgenology* 1983; **14**: 1027–33.

10. Schwab SJ, Hlatky MA, Pieper KS *et al.* Contrast nephrotoxicity. A randomized, controlled trial of a nonionic and an ionic radiographic contrast agent. *New England Journal of Medicine* 1989; **320**: 149–53.

11. Powe NR, Steinberg EP, Erickson JR *et al.* Contrast medium-induced adverse reactions: economic outcome. *Radiology* 1988; **169**: 163–8.

12. Older RA, Korobkin M, Cleeve DM, Schaaf R, Thompson W. Contrast-induced acute renal failure: persistent nephrogram as clue to early detection. *American Journal of Roentgenology* 1980; **134**: 339–42.

13. D'Elia JA, Gleason RE, Alday M *et al.* Nephrotoxicity from angiographic contrast material. A prospective study. *American Journal of Medicine* 1982; **72**: 719–25.

14. Harkonen S, Kjellstrand CM. Exacerbation of diabetic renal failure following intravenous pyelography. *American Journal of Medicine* 1977; **63**: 939–46.

15. Gomes AS, Baker JD, Martin-Paredero V *et al.* Acute renal dysfunction after major arteriography. *American Journal of Roentgenology* 1985; **145**: 1249–53.

16. Byrd L, Sherman RL. Radiocontrast-induced acute renal failure: a clinical and pathophysiologic review. *Medicine* 1979; **58**: 270–9.

17. Carvallo A, Rakowski TA, Argy WP, Schreiner GE. Acute renal failure following drip-infusion pyelography. *American Journal of Medicine* 1978; **65**: 38–45.

18. Cramer BC, Parfrey PS, Hutchinson TA *et al.* Renal function following infusion of radiologic contrast material. A prospective, controlled study. *Archives of Internal Medicine* 1985; **145**: 87–9.

19. Parfrey PS, Griffiths SM, Barrett BJ *et al.* Contrast material-induced renal failure in patients with diabetes mellitus, renal insufficiency, or both. *New England Journal of Medicine* 1989; **320**: 143–9.

20. Solomon R, Werner G, Mann D, D'Elia J, Silva P. Effects of saline, mannitol, and furosemide on acute decreases in renal function induced by radiocontrast agents. *New England Journal of Medicine* 1994; **331**: 1416–20.

21. Barrett BJ, Carlisle EJ. Meta-analysis of the relative nephrotoxicity of high- and low-osmolality iodinated contrast media. *Radiology* 1993; **188**: 171–8.

22. Rudnick MR, Goldfarb S, Wexler L *et al.* Nephrotoxicity of ionic and nonionic contrast media in 1196 patients: a randomized trial. *Kidney International* 1995; **46**: 254–61.

23. Thomsen HS, Dorph S, Larsen S *et al.* Urine profiles and kidney histology after intravenous injection of ionic and nonionic radiologic and magnetic resonance contrast media in normal rats. *Academic Radiology* 1994; **1**: 128–35.

24. Frennby B, Sterner G, Almen T, Hagstam K-E, Hultberg B, Jacobsson L. The use of iohexol clearance to determine GFR in patients with severe chronic renal failure – a comparison between different clearance techniques. *Clinical Nephrology* 1995; **43**: 35–46.

25. Sterner G, Frennby B, Hultberg B, Almen T. Iohexol clearance for GFR determination in renal failure – single or multiple plasma sampling. *Nephrology, Dialysis, Transplantation* 1996; **11**: 521–5.

26. Prince MR, Arnoldus C, Frisoli JK. Nephrotoxicity of high-dose gadolinium compared with iodinated contrast. *Journal of Magnetic Resonance Imaging* 1996; **1**: 162–6.

27. Joffe P, Thomsen HS, Meusel M. Pharmacokinetics of gadodiamide injection in patients with severe renal insufficiency and patients undergoing hemodialysis or continuous ambulatory hemodialysis. *Academic Radiology* 1998; **5**: 491–502.

Case studies: adult emergency radiology situations

Bernard F. King Jr and Karl N. Krecke

Case studies

Case 1

Background   A 23-year-old woman with a history of myasthenia gravis was having a contrast-enhanced chest CT examination using conventional high-osmolality ionic-contrast material. She experienced severe muscle weakness, inability to swallow, weak respiration and inability to talk.

Management   We closely monitored her vital signs, particularly her respiratory status.

Learning point   IV contrast material may precipitate a myasthenia gravis crisis. It may be necessary to provide respiratory support, from supplementary oxygen to intubation, until the myasthenia crisis has passed.

Case 2

Background   A 71-year-old woman was having an abdominal CT examination. Approximately 2 min after injection of 150 mL of high-osmolality contrast material, the patient complained of feeling unwell, nausea and tingling.

Management   The nurse noticed that the patient was becoming pale and measured her blood pressure, which was 60/30 mmHg. The patient became unresponsive. There was some difficulty in locating the radiologist. The patient then appeared to have seizure activity. At that point, another radiologist was located and arrived at the scene. Intravenous fluids were started. The patient stopped breathing, and the Code team was called. Mouth-to-mask ventilation with supplementary oxygen was given for about 1 min before the patient began breathing on her own. Shortly thereafter, the Code team arrived and ordered epinephrine (1:10 000) 3 mL IV, Benadryl® 50 mg IV and Solu-Cortef® 100 mg IV. Several minutes later, a dopamine (800 μg/ml) drip was started because of persistent hypotension. At some point during the administration of these medications, the nurse and physician noticed erythema, a few hives on the face, and puffy eyelids. The patient was transferred to the emergency room and was then hospitalized. The patient was discharged 2 days later in good condition.

Learning points

1 The radiologist responsible for the patient should have been immediately available or should have arranged coverage by a colleague.

2 A competent physician, preferably the attending radiologist, should be immediately available for at least 5 min after the injection of contrast media. This might have allowed more prompt diagnosis and institution of appropriate therapy for this patient.

3 *No pulse was recorded.* Although the pulse rate may be difficult to obtain in a patient who is hypotensive, it can be of critical importance in differentiating the specific therapy for a patient with hypotension and tachycardia from that for a patient with a vasovagal reaction (hypotension plus bradycardia).

Case 3

Background A 77-year-old woman was having a CT exam to evaluate a new lung mass. She had significant cardiac disease with history of dysrhythmias. She was very anxious from the start of the examination and described a sense of claustrophobia. Nonionic, lower-osmolality contrast material was used, and she remained anxious and somewhat agitated during the course of the examination. At the conclusion of fast scanning, she wanted to get out of the scanner and sit up. Her blood pressure measured at that time was considerably elevated (180/120 mmHg). She then described some shortness of breath.

Management Oxygen was given by mask. Diffuse crackles were heard in the mid and lower lungs on auscultatory examination, although there was no evidence of wheezing. Previous chest X-ray had shown the lungs to be clear. The first images processed from the CT examination showed a diffuse increase in interstitial markings, which was a new development from the chest X-ray and raised suspicion of pulmonary edema. The patient continued to have elevated blood pressure in the range 200/140 mmHg and started to describe a feeling of chest heaviness. At that point, a Code was called, and the patient was given nitroglycerin 0.4 mg sublingually. As the Code team arrived, she began coughing frothy, pink sputum. At that point, the patient was given morphine and furosemide IV for pulmonary edema and increased blood pressure. She was transported from the department to the emergency room.

Learning points

1 We could have been more suspicious of the patient's anxiety and agitation and not attributed it solely to claustrophobia.

2 We could have taken a blood pressure measurement earlier in the examination.

3 Although pulmonary edema is a relatively uncommon complication of contrast material administration, it is a very serious reaction, and it is important to recognize it early. The exact etiology is uncertain, and it is usually not a direct effect of the volume of contrast medium injected. Early involvement of the Code team and transfer from the department to the emergency room are very important in the management of such patients. The timely use of furosemide can be very useful in controlling the symptoms.

Case 4

Background An elderly man had a CT-guided biopsy of his renal mass. Approximately 15 min after the procedure, the nurse recorded a blood pressure of 100/70 mmHg with a pulse of 64 beats/min. Prior to biopsy, the blood pressure was 140/80 mmHg with a pulse of 70 beats/min. The blood pressure was taken again and determined to be 82/60 mmHg with a pulse of 64 beats/min. The patient was asymptomatic and not diaphoretic.

Management The patient's legs were elevated and IV fluids were started. He continued to be asymptomatic. The blood pressure continued at 82/60 mmHg with a pulse of 64 beats/min. The patient was then given 0.5 mg atropine IV. Several minutes later, his blood pressure was 98/68 mmHg with a pulse of 68 beats/min. Approximately 30 min later, the blood pressure was 82/60 mmHg with a pulse of 62 beats/min. IV fluids continued to be given (over 1L at this point). The patient continued to be asymptomatic.

Repeat CT scan through the biopsy region was negative for hemorrhage.

A blood-pressure cuff was placed on the opposite arm while the patient was being moved into the CT gantry. This time the blood pressure was 130/80 mmHg. The patient then recalled that he had been told about a blood-pressure discrepancy in his upper extremities. There was no note on the chart concerning this.

Learning points

1 We should have questioned the blood pressure readings in the face of a completely asymptomatic patient.

2 Be consistent with the site of blood pressure measurement.

3 Consider technical factors, normal variants, and coincidental pathologies when the patient's symptoms and clinical signs do not match.

Case 5

Background I was called into the ultrasound room because the patient had 'turned blue'.

Management The nurse who accompanied the patient to the radiology department had started chest compression. That left only one thing for me – the mouth-to-mouth part. I looked around the room for the mask that covers the patient's mouth and could not find it. Therefore, I had to resort to the conventional mouth-to-mouth technique. At this point, the ICU nurse noticed the plastic mask attached to the wall, knew how to assemble and use it, and offered to exchange places with me.

Learning point   I wish I had taken a few moments before a Code situation to become familiar with the mask and its normal location, in a nonurgent situation. These masks are placed within plastic packs that are ideal for emergency medical teams to carry, but the mask needs to be removed from the plastic container and assembled before it can be used. I urge everyone to learn how to use this mask before the need to use it emergently arises.

Case 6

Background   I was called to the CT examination room because the patient was 'not feeling good' and was hypotensive.

Management   The nurse and the other physician tending the patient stated that the patient did not feel good, but his blood pressure was fairly normal (110/60mmHg). As I entered the room, the patient was losing consciousness and had no palpable pulse or blood pressure. Fortunately, an IV had been started, and I instructed the nurse to give the patient 0.5 mL (50 μg) of 1:10 000 dilution epinephrine IV.

Prior to the administration of epinephrine, the patient was dusky in appearance, clammy, cold and unconscious. Immediately following administration, the patient became pink and conscious. In addition, we could immediately palpate a pulse and his blood pressure returned to 120/80 mmHg. The patient was then transferred to the local emergency room for further monitoring.

Learning points

1   At the time when the patient became unresponsive, it was unclear what was going on. We did not know whether the patient was vasovagal with a low heart rate or in shock from cardiovascular collapse with a high heart rate. What was clear was that something needed to be done immediately, otherwise the patient would go into cardiac arrest.

2   A small dose (e.g. 0.5 mL) of 1:10 000 dilution IV epinephrine is appropriate therapy for profound hypotension in the context of contrast administration. Vasopressor administration in low doses is appropriate in the initial treatment of profound vagal reaction prior to administration of atropine.

Case 7

Background   I was called into the urography room because the patient felt light-headed.

Management The patient's blood pressure was approximately 90/60 mmHg. He was an African-American who, other than feeling slightly lightheaded, was otherwise comfortable. His heart rate was approximately 80–90 beats/min. IV fluids were started, and the patient's legs were elevated. His blood pressure responded to the IV fluids, and after 1 L of fluid the blood pressure was 105/70 mmHg. The heart rate was still 80 beats/min. At this point in time (approximately 30 min after the beginning of the reaction) we decided to turn off the IV fluids. As soon as we did this, the patient's blood pressure dropped down to 80/60 mmHg again. His blood pressure was brought back up with another liter of IV fluid and again the patient reported feeling fine. One hour and 2 L of IV fluids later, it was clear that the patient was not stable enough to be released because of his dependence on IV fluids to maintain blood pressure. At this time, the diagnosis of diffuse erythema was made by blanching the skin on the back of his hand and arm. This was difficult to detect because of the patient's dark skin color. After a third liter of IV fluids, the patient's blood pressure was still hovering around 90–100 mmHg systolic, and at this point the decision was made to send him to the emergency room. In the emergency room, the patient received corticosteroids, diphenhydramine, and an additional 1 to 2 L of IV fluids, and spent the night in the emergency-room.

The emergency-room physician was upset that we had not administered any medications to the patient in the face of persistent hypotension and erythema.

Learning points

1 In African-American people or others with dark skin color, diffuse erythema may be difficult to detect.

2 If therapy requires more than 1 or 2 L of IV fluid to maintain a patient's blood pressure, it is time to move the patient quickly to an emergency room for more intensive care.

3 Small doses of IV epinephrine (1.0 mL or less of 1:10 000 dilution) should also have been considered when the patient failed to respond to fluid therapy. Epinephrine is very effective in treating diffuse cutaneous and vasodilating reactions.

4 If a serious reaction (erythema and hypotension) is persisting, and after the situation is under control and the patient's condition has stabilized, it is appropriate to also administer an IV antihistamine such as diphenhydramine and IV corticosteroids. Steroids and antihistamines however are unlikely to benefit the patient substantially until several hours after they are administered.

Case 8

Background A 70-year-old woman was undergoing an angiogram of the lower extremity vessels with ionic low-osmolality contrast medium (LOCM). Following the injection, the patient complained of increasing shortness of breath. Auscultation of the lungs revealed crackles at both bases. Her blood pressure was 240/124 mmHg. The patient had a significant history of atherosclerotic disease, chronic atrial fibrillation, chronic hypertension, diabetes mellitus, rheumatic valvular disease resulting in moderate mitral stenosis, and moderate aortic stenosis with a minimal amount of ischemic heart disease.

Management Despite the immediate administration of two IV doses of furosemide (40 mg), 5 mg of nifedipine sublingually, and 10 mg of hydrazaline IV, the patient's blood pressure and shortness of breath continued to worsen. She was emergently transferred to the cardiac intensive-care unit, at which time she was placed on a nitroglycerin drip for afterload reduction and blood pressure control. The patient was given 100 per cent oxygen by mask. Despite this, O_2 saturations remained less than 90 per cent. Chest X-ray revealed perihilar pulmonary edema.

The patient was intubated and placed on positive ventilatory pressures. At the time of intubation, pink frothy sputum was aspirated from the airways consistent with pulmonary edema. An emergent cardiac echo was performed and revealed normal left ventricular size and function, with an ejection fraction of 65 per cent. There was mild mitral regurgitation and aortic regurgitation on the echo.

The patient gradually responded to lowering of her blood pressure and subsequent improvement of her pulmonary edema and was extubated approximately 36 h after the angiogram. Additional medications included hydrocortisone and diphenhydramine to counter any histamine-mediated processes.

Learning points

1 Contrast medium-induced pulmonary edema is a well-known and well-recognized adverse contrast reaction. It appears to occur equally often with nonionic and ionic agents. The hypertensive reaction may have been the precipitating cause of the decompensation of the left ventricle which resulted in pulmonary edema.

2 Pulmonary edema caused by contrast media is a very serious and life-threatening reaction. Therapy consisting of high-flow oxygen, IV furosemide and morphine sulfate is indicated for prompt treatment. Since most patients with pulmonary edema do not respond rapidly to therapy, prompt transportation to an emergency room or intensive-care unit is paramount.

Case 9

Background A 53-year-old woman underwent an aortogram utilizing ionic high-osmolality contrast medium (HOCM) without complications. Approximately 20 min later, nausea and vomiting occurred immediately after an angiogram of the lower extremities utilizing ionic LOCM. During the nausea and vomiting the patient's face became diffusely red, but there was no evidence of diffuse body erythema. At this time the patient was noted to have a normal blood pressure and heart rate. Approximately 2 min later the patient began to complain of difficulty in breathing and became quite agitated. Her lungs sounded clear with no wheezing. An arterial blood-pressure line that was in place revealed a precipitous drop in systolic blood pressure.

Management   At this time, 1 mg of epinephrine (1:10 000 dilution) in a 10-mL vial was administered IV slowly in 1-mL (0.1 mg) increments. Despite this, the blood pressure continued to drop and became undetectable. A second dose of 1 mg of epinephrine (1:10 000, 1-mL increments) was given IV. A full Code was started and the patient was immediately intubated. The patient developed an agonal rhythm and, despite further injections of IV epinephrine, there was no response in heart rate or blood pressure. Fluoroscopic examination during the Code revealed no evidence of pulmonary edema in the chest. A temporary pacemaker was placed without response. A short injection of contrast into the main pulmonary artery during the Code revealed no evidence of a pulmonary embolism. Despite all of these measures, the patient died. Post-mortem examination revealed an extensive myocardial infarction due to an acute occlusion of the left main coronary artery.

Learning points

1 Acute onset of nausea and vomiting is a relatively common physiologic response to contrast material injection. However, a delayed onset of nausea and vomiting should be viewed as a potential sign of a more severe event.

2 Myocardial infarction can be a sequela of contrast medium administration. Despite all efforts, with immediate response by anesthesia and cardiology personnel, this patient's myocardial infarction could not be reversed.

Case 10

Background   A 40-year-old man was undergoing cerebral angiography for a possible diagnosis of CNS vasculitis. Following the first injection of low-osmolality nonionic iodinated contrast material, the patient's blood pressure drifted down to 100/60 mmHg, with an increase in heart rate to 100–110 beats/min. The drapes were pulled back, revealing diffuse erythema over the patient's trunk and extremities.

Management   Intravenous fluids were increased, and 1 mL of 1:10 000 dilution epinephrine was given IV. The patient's blood pressure continued to fall to approximately 90/50 mmHg with a heart rate of 120 beats/min. The patient was minimally symptomatic. A second dose of 1 mL of 1:10 000 dilution epinephrine was given, and the patient's blood pressure responded promptly, rising to 150/80 mmHg. Steroids and diphenhydramine were also administered at this point. The patient was now asymptomatic. After a few minutes, a third dose of epinephrine was given 'to stop the cascade' and to forestall and recurrence of hypotension. The patient's blood pressure promptly increased to 240/110 mmHg. He initially complained of headache, and then he became aphasic. The hypertension was transient, and within a few minutes the aphasia cleared and his blood pressure normalized. Postprocedural head CT was negative, and the erythema had resolved. The patient was admitted for observation and discharged the following day.

Learning point   Epinephrine is the drug of choice to combat severe anaphylactoid reaction. However, it is a very potent adrenergic agent and the dosage should be titrated to effect. It is not a drug to be given prophylactically. The extra dose given in this case was not appropriate in a clinically stable patient.

Case 11

Background   The radiologist was called to see a patient undergoing a CT examination of the head for 'spells'. The patient had received iodinated contrast material and was now gesturing that she was having trouble breathing – grasping her chest and neck with her hands. The radiologist queried the patient, who continued to grasp urgently at her neck and chest without speaking.

Management   The radiologist then administered 3 mL of 1:10 000 dilution epinephrine IV to treat presumed airway compromise secondary to anaphylactoid reaction. The patient promptly sat up, speaking rapidly and clearly in Spanish. She had tachycardia with increased blood pressure and was agitated. Her breath sounds were clear and now hyperdynamic. Her husband later scolded the radiologist, saying that his wife had shown exactly the same reaction following administration of contrast material in her native country and was told never to have contrast material again. By the time the whole scenario had ended, it was evident that the radiologist had treated a panic attack with IV epinephrine.

Learning points

1 Diagnose before beginning treatment. The radiologist did not check breath sounds, blood pressure or pulse prior to administration of a large dose of epinephrine.

2 Panic attacks can mimic more serious anaphylactoid reactions, with symptoms of respiratory distress, chest pain and unconsciousness.

3 If epinephrine is indicated in the setting of legitimate anaphylactoid reaction, one should begin with a smaller dose (e.g. 1 mL of 1:10 000 dilution) and administer it slowly, titrating to effect.

12 Case studies: cardiac dysrhythmias

Thomas F. Bugliosi, William H. Bush Jr and Geoffrey S. Ferguson

The following case studies are examples of various cardiac dysrhythmias. Correct interpretation is the first step but, more importantly, remember that you need to treat the patient, not the monitor.

For many abnormal rhythms you will have time to evaluate the overall situation and obtain assistance or consultation. For others (e.g. ventricular fibrillation, pulseless ventricular tachycardia) you must act quickly and decisively with prompt defibrillation.

Case studies

Case 1

During angiography of the legs, your patient complains of a mild increase in shortness of breath. You check the monitor and see this rhythm:

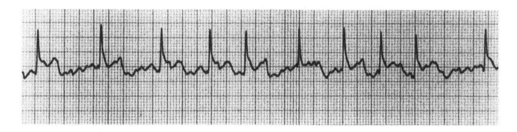

What is your diagnosis?

- (a) Normal sinus rhythm
- (b) Atrial fibrillation
- (c) Ventricular fibrillation
- (d) Ventricular tachycardia

Case 2

When you connect the monitor to the patient at the beginning of a CT-guided lung biopsy, you discover this rhythm:

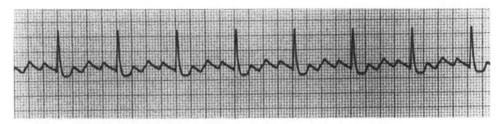

What is your diagnosis?

    (a) Ventricular tachycardia
    (b) Normal sinus rhythm
    (c) Atrial flutter
    (d) Pulseless electrical activity (PEA)

Case 3

During abscess drainage in CT, you observe this rhythm on the monitor. The patient notices 'something' but cannot describe it well.

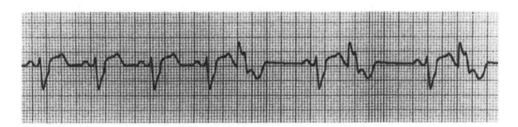

What is your diagnosis?

    (a) Normal sinus rhythm
    (b) Premature atrial contraction (PAC)
    (c) Normal sinus rhythm with premature ventricular contractions (PVC)
    (d) Ventricular fibrillation

Case 4

During a CT scan of a patient with lower leg pain, the technologist calls you because the cardiac rhythm has changed. You check the monitor and see this rhythm:

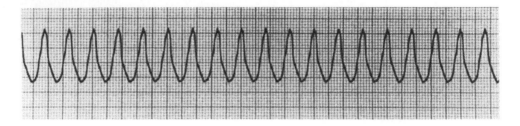

What is your diagnosis?

  (a) Ventricular fibrillation
  (b) Ventricular tachycardia
  (c) Atrial tachycardia
  (d) Pulseless electrical activity (PEA)

Case 5

During a CT scan, at the end of injection, the patient becomes unresponsive. You check for a pulse and find none. You call a 'Code' and take a 'quick look' with the defibrillator paddles. This shows you the following rhythm:

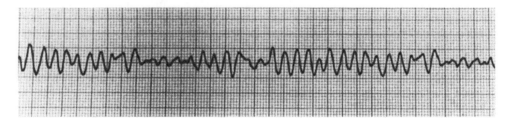

What is your diagnosis?

  (a) Ventricular fibrillation
  (b) Ventricular tachycardia
  (c) Atrial tachycardia
  (d) Atrial fibrillation

Answers

Case 1 (b, atrial fibrillation)

Atrial fibrillation is characterized by an irregularly irregular (chaotic) ventricular response (ventricular rate is often 160–180 beats/min). The atrial rate is so fast that no organized P waves are identifiable (atrial rate is in fact 400–700 beats/min).

Case 2 (c, atrial flutter)

Atrial flutter is believed to be caused by a re-entry phenomenon at the atrial level. The atrial rate is usually about 300 beats/min and appears as a 'saw tooth' pattern in lead II. The AV node often blocks down in an even manner (2:1, 4:1), giving a ventricular rate of 150 or 75 beats/min.

Case 3 (c, normal sinus rhythm with premature ventricular contractions (PVC)

Premature ventricular contraction is an abnormal depolarization that arises in either ventricle and causes simultaneous ventricular depolarization resulting in a wide ($\geq$ 0.125), bizarre-appearing QRS complex and T wave. It occurs 'prematurely' relative to the patient's regular QRS sequence. In Case 3, the PVCs are unifocal.

Case 4 (b, ventricular tachycardia)

Ventricular tachycardia is defined as three or more beats of ventricular origin occurring in a row, at a rate in excess of 100 beats/min. The QRS complexes are wide, the rate is usually regular, and there may be AV dissociation. Ventricular tachycardia may produce a stable, unstable or 'arrested' patient. Ventricular tachycardia is always a medical emergency because decompensation may occur and ventricular fibrillation can develop.

Case 5 (a, ventricular fibrillation)

Ventricular fibrillation is a life-threatening, non-conducting rhythm. It is the most commonly encountered rhythm in out-of-hospital arrest and is the reason why early defibrillation has been emphasized in the emergency medical response system. Without correction, the likelihood of survival decreases with each passing minute. Ventricular fibrillation is characterized by a disorganized rhythm that is too fast to count. No definite P waves, QRS, ST segment or T wave can be seen. Immediate recognition and defibrillation are mandatory.

Discussion

Atrial tachycardias   For paroxysmal supraventricular tachycardia (PSVT), you may try vagal manuevers (e.g. valsalva) or adenosine (6 mg) IV push. If the rhythm is clearly atrial fibrillation or atrial flutter, medication options include beta-blockers, though synchronized cardioversion may be necessary. Consultation with the primary-care physician is suggested.

Premature ventricular contraction (PVC)   Occasional PVCs in the asymptomatic patient without suspected heart disease do not require treatment. If the PVCs are symptomatic and prompt treatment is necessary, IV lidocaine is the drug of choice.

Asystole   The straight line on an ECG indicates complete absence of ventricular activity. There is no depolarization and no ventricular contraction. Asystole may occur as a primary event or as the end-result of failed cardiac resuscitation. In either case, successful resuscitation from asystole is very rare.

Pulseless electrical activity (PEA)   (previously termed electromechanical dissociation or EMD) is present when the ECG shows activity but there is no detectable pulse and the patient is unresponsive. There may be an underlying cause such as hypoxia, hypotension or hypocalcemia that is potentially correctable. It may represent a failing myocardium. PEA is treated in the same way as asystole.

Cardiac arrest
The priorities in caring for cardiac arrest concern oxygenation and circulation. Early defibrillation for ventricular fibrillation and pulseless ventricular tachycardia are mandatory.

1   Establish non-responsiveness/apnea/pulselessness.

2   Activate the emergency response system.

3   Begin cardiopulmonary resuscitation:
   * primary emergency worker begins artificial ventilation using airway and bag-valve-mask (high-flow oxygen) and suction as needed;
   * second emergency worker begins chest compression.

4   As soon as possible attach the cardiac monitor.

5   If the rhythm is pulseless ventricular tachycardia or ventricular fibrillation, charge the defibrillator to 200 joules and defibrillate the patient, ensuring first that no personnel are in contact with the patient or stretcher/bed.

6   If there is no change in rhythm, defibrillate with 300 joules.

7   If there is no change in rhythm, defibrillate with 360 joules.

8   If, after three defibrillation attempts, there is no change or if the rhythm is not ventricular fibrillation or pulseless ventricular tachycardia, resume CPR.

9 Intravenously, give 1 mg epinephrine (10 mL of 1:10 000 solution IV). Continue cardiopulmonary resuscitation to circulate the drug.

10 If the rhythm remains pulseless ventricular tachycardia or ventricular fibrillation, defibrillate again with 360 joules.

11 If the rhythm is unchanged, give 1 mg of atropine.

12 Continue CPR to circulate the drug.

References

Emergency Care Committee, American Hospital Association. Guidelines for cardiopulmonary resusitation and emergency cardiac care. *Journal of the American Medical Association* 1992; **268**: 2135–302.

Grauer E, Cavallaro D. *Advanced cardiac life support (Volumes I and II)*. New York: Mosby, 1993.

13 Case studies: contrast nephrotoxicity

Henrik S. Thomsen and William H. Bush Jr

Introduction

The radiologist performs several injections of contrast media daily. However, from time to time one encounters a patient for whom intravascular contrast medium is inappropriate due to an increased risk of contrast-induced nephrotoxicity. In this chapter, typical clinical situations are presented with multiple-choice questions, followed by an explanation for the best answers in relation to the *kidney*.

Case studies

Case 1
A 70-year-old man has diabetes mellitus and his serum creatinine level is 200 μmol/L (2.3 mg/dL). The clinician requests intravenous urography because of a new finding of hematuria.

What action would you take?

   (a) Proceed with the requested intravenous urogram
   (b) Postpone the examination
   (c) MRI
   (d) Ultrasonography
   (e) CT without and with IV contrast medium
   (f) Retrograde pyelography in conjunction with cystoscopy

Case 2
A 70-year-old man has diabetes mellitus and his serum creatinine level is 200 μmol/L (2.3 mg/dL). The clinician suspects a brain tumor and requests a CT scan of the brain with intravenous contrast.

What action would you take?

   (a) Proceed with the requested contrast-enhanced brain CT
   (b) Postpone the examination
   (c) MRI
   (d) Cerebral arteriography

Case 3

A 70-year-old man with diabetes mellitus and a serum creatinine level of 530 μmol/L (6.0 mg/dL) is on chronic hemodialysis. The patient has known treated brain metastases, and a brain CT examination is requested for followup. The clinician prefers CT due to cost and expediency.

What action would you take?

    (a) Proceed with the requested contrast-enhanced brain CT
    (b) MRI
    (c) Radionuclide brain scan

Case 4

A 50-year-old woman has verified analgesic nephropathy. Her serum creatinine level is 500 μmol/L (5.7 mg/dL). Intravenous urography is requested because of clinical suspicion of obstruction.

What action would you take?

    (a) Proceed with the requested intravenous urogram
    (b) Postpone the examination
    (c) MRI
    (d) Ultrasonography
    (e) CT without and with IV contrast
    (f) Radionuclide imaging of the kidneys and collecting systems
    (g) Retrograde pyelography

Case 5

A 60-year-old woman who takes nonsteroidal anti-inflammatory drugs (NSAIDs) for arthritis is admitted with a swollen leg. Her serum creatinine level on admission is 150 μmol/L (1.7 mg/dL). Due to clinical suspicion of deep vein thrombophlebitis, peripheral venography is requested.

What action would you take?

    (a) Proceed with the requested venography
    (b) Postpone the examination
    (c) MRI
    (d) Ultrasonography

Case 6

A 40-year-old man is admitted with renal colic. An intravenous urogram is requested to verify the presence of an obstructing stone. The patient has had several episodes of renal colic and his serum creatinine level is known to be stable at 150 μmol/L (1.7 mg/dl). He takes no medication.

What action would you take?

(a) Proceed with the requested intravenous urogram
(b) Postpone the examination
(c) MRI
(d) Ultrasonography
(e) CT of abdomen and pelvis without contrast medium
(f) CT of abdomen and pelvis without and with contrast medium
(g) Radionuclide imaging of the kidneys and collecting systems

Case 7

A 65-year-old man has known bladder cancer close to the vesico-ureteral junctions. His serum creatinine level has remained unchanged during the past year at 150 μmol/L (1.7 mg/dL). Due to jaundice, CT scanning of the liver is requested.

What action would you take?

(a) Proceed with the requested contrast-enhanced abdominal CT
(b) Postpone the examination
(c) MRI
(d) Ultrasonography
(e) Radionuclide imaging of the liver

Case 8

A 65 year-old-man with diabetes mellitus is referred for coronary arteriography because of cardiac ischemia. His serum creatinine level is 90 μmol/L (1.0 mg/dL).

What action would you take?

(a) Proceed with the requested angiography
(b) Postpone the examination
(c) MRI
(d) Radionuclide imaging of the heart

Case 9

A 60-year-old woman with myelomatosis (multiple myeloma) has an abnormal chest radiograph. CT scanning of the mediastinum is requested. The patient's serum creatinine level has been stable at 150 μmol/L (1.7 mg/dL) for the past 6 months.

What action would you take?

(a) Proceed with chest CT using IV contrast medium
(b) Postpone the examination
(c) Chest CT without contrast medium
(d) Chest MRI

Case 10

A 77-year-old woman with noticeable arteriosclerosis underwent hysterectomy 3 days ago. Her urinary output is now low and her serum creatinine level is increasing.

The gynecologist suspects surgical damage to a ureter and requests intravenous urography.

What action would you take?

   (a) Proceed with urography and consider trying to increase the washout of contrast medium with furosemide
   (b) Postpone the examination
   (c) MRI of the abdomen and pelvis
   (d) Ultrasonography
   (e) CT of the abdomen and pelvis without and with contrast medium
   (f) Radionuclide imaging of the kidneys and collecting systems

Case 11

A 65-year-old woman has diabetes mellitus and a serum creatinine level of 90 μmol/L (1.0 mg/dL). To complete preoperative evaluation for her verified cancer of the colon, the surgeons request contrast-enhanced CT scanning of the liver.

What action would you take?

   (a) Proceed with the requested liver CT
   (b) Postpone the examination
   (c) MRI of the liver
   (d) Ultrasonography
   (e) Radionuclide imaging of the liver

Answers

It should be emphasized that the answers given below are all worded in relation to the *kidney*. In some instances you may choose to perform a different examination because of local availability or preference for a different diagnostic strategy. There may also be cases where, based on the initially obtained unenhanced examination, you do not believe that you need to continue with an enhanced examination because you have already obtained adequate diagnostic information. *No priority of answers is intended in the listing of several correct responses.*

Case 1: (c, d, f)
The abnormal serum creatinine level indicates that the patient has diabetic nephropathy. This places the patient in the highest-risk group for developing contrast-induced nephropathy.[2,7] Therefore, the intravascular administration of iodinated contrast medium should be avoided.

Case 2: (c)
As in Case 1, this patient has an increased serum creatinine level, indicating diabetic nephropathy. Therefore, if possible, the patient should be referred for MRI of

the brain, in which a much lower dose of contrast medium (gadolinium agent) is used.[3] The molar dose of gadolinium chelates used for MRI of the brain is about one-ninth of the dose of iodinated contrast media used for CT of the brain. The higher the molar dose, the higher the risk.

In fact, Case 1 and Case 2 refer to the same patient. The patient was admitted with hematuria and an intravenous urogram was requested. Before it was carried out, the urogram was cancelled because the referring clinician considered it risky to administer contrast medium to this patient with diabetic nephropathy. However, in the following week the same clinician requested a CT examination of the brain. It is important to remember that, regardless of which organ is being examined with contrast medium, the contrast is excreted from the body through the kidneys, and the risk of contrast-induced nephropathy is independent of the organ examined.[2]

Case 3 (a)

In the patient with chronic nephropathy who is already commited to hemodialysis, one may proceed with contrast-enhanced CT of organs other than the kidneys. Further renal damage is not an issue. If parenchymal phase imaging is all that is necessary (i.e. arterial and venous phases are not necessary), one can lower the total iodine load (a reduced amount of contrast medium is given for the examination) because the effective load of iodine will be higher due to lack of kidney filtration. However, if the patient still has enough minimal renal function to allow treatment by peritoneal dialysis rather than hemodialysis, nephrotoxic contrast media should not be used in order to avoid further loss of renal function and subsequent commitment of the patient to hemodialysis. For that patient, MRI should be used.

Case 4 (c, f, g)

The serum creatinine concentration is above the level at which an adequate diagnostic urogram can be obtained. Furthermore, the risk of causing further deterioration in kidney function is substantial. Therefore, another examination should be used. Ultrasonography may give false-negative results because the pelvo-ureteral system is dilated from previous passage of sloughed papilla, or extremely poor kidney function may not distend the obstructed upper urinary tract.

Case 5 (b, d)

It is known that nonsteroidal anti-inflammatory drugs (NSAIDs) can cause renal dysfunction, and concomitant administration of contrast media might cause further deterioration. Therefore, ultrasonography should be performed and the requested venography should be postponed or cancelled. If renal function improves after ceasing administration of NSAIDs, venography can be performed when the serum creatinine level has normalized.

Case 6 (a)

The patient's renal dysfunction has been stable for 1 year and the probable cause is obstructive nephropathy. Obstructive nephropathy is not considered to increase the risk of contrast medium-induced nephrotoxicity.[2] Therefore one can proceed with the intravenous urogram, so long as one ensures that the patient is well hydrated. A CT examination without contrast medium is also an excellent method of demonstrating calculi, including those composed of urate.[4]

Case 7 (a)
The patient's increased serum creatinine level is most probably due to obstructive nephropathy. Therefore, as discussed in Case 6, one can hydrate the patient well and proceed with a contrast-enhanced CT examination of the liver.

Case 8 (a)
The patient has diabetes mellitus, but the serum creatinine level indicates that diabetic nephropathy is not present. Diabetes mellitus *without* nephropathy does not put the patient in the high-risk group for developing contrast-induced nephropathy.[1,2,5,6] Therefore one can proceed with cardiac angiography.

Case 9 (a)
During the 1950s, 1960s and 1970s, myelomatosis (multiple myeloma) was considered to be an absolute contraindication for administration of contrast media. More recent investigations have shown that hydration of the patient greatly reduces the risk.[7] Therefore one can proceed with administration of contrast medium if it is appropriate for the diagnostic workup and the patient is adequately hydrated.

Case 10 (c, d, e, f)
The patient's kidney function is deteriorating. The patient has arteriosclerosis and is probably dehydrated after the surgery. The risk of causing further deterioration in kidney function as a result of contrast medium injection is high. Furthermore, the contrast medium (as well as furosemide) may cause further dehydration. Due to the arteriosclerosis, the patient may be unable to compensate for dehydration and the amount of contrast medium excreted per minute may not be sufficient to detect leakage from a ureter injury. Therefore, another approach in which a contrast medium is not administered should be chosen, and radionuclide scintigraphy is often effective in demonstrating a ureter leak.

Case 11 (a)
As in Case 8, one may proceed with the requested contrast-enhanced examination. The serum creatinine level does not indicate the presence of diabetic nephropathy. Diabetes mellitus without nephropathy does not put the patient in the high-risk group for developing contrast-induced nephropathy.[5,6]

Measures to prevent contrast-induced nephropathy

Contrast-induced nephropathy cannot be avoided altogether, but the risk to individual patients can be reduced. Screening of patients for risk factors, especially diabetes mellitus with renal dysfunction, is very important. The most effective measures to prevent its occurrence are as follows:[2,8,9]

1 Adequate hydration. Extracellular volume expansion is achieved with oral fluids or intravenous fluids (saline) securing a diuresis of > 1 mL/min. This can be obtained by administering 100 mL/h of fluid starting 4 h before the contrast examination, and continuing IV fluids at that rate for 24 h after the administration of a contrast medium. Of course the rate is modified in the clinical situation of heart failure.

2 Nonionic, low-osmolality contrast media should always be used for a patient at risk of contrast-induced nephrotoxicity (e.g. a diabetic with evidence of renal dysfunction).

3 It is advisable that the interval between contrast-enhanced examinations should be at least 48 h.

4 Concomitant use of nephrotoxic drugs should be avoided.

References

1. Berns AS. Nephrotoxicity of contrast media. *Kidney International* 1989; **36**: 730–40.

2. Thomsen HS. Contrast nephropathy. *Current Opinion in Radiology* 1990; **2**: 793–802.

3. Thomsen HS, Dorph S, Larsen S *et al.* Urine profiles and kidney histology after intravenous injection of ionic and nonionic radiologic and magnetic resonance contrast media in normal rats. *Academic Radiology* 1994; **2**: 128–35.

4. Smith RC, Rosenfield AT, Choe KA *et al.* Acute flank pain: comparison of noncontrast-enhanced CT and intravenous urography. *Radiology* 1995; **194**: 789–94.

5. Barret BJ, Carlisle EJ. Meta-analysis of the relative nephrotoxicity of high- and low-osmolality iodinated contrast media. *Radiology* 1993; **188**: 171–8.

6. Rudnick MR, Goldfarb S, Wexler L *et al.* Nephrotoxicity of ionic and non-ionic contrast media in 1196 patients: a randomized trial. *Kidney International* 1995; **46**: 254–61.

7. McCarthy CS, Becker JA. Multiple myeloma and contrast media. *Radiology* 1992; **183**: 519–21.

8. Solomon R, Werner G, Mann D *et al.* Effects of saline, mannitol and furosemide on acute decreases in renal function induced by radiocontrast agents. *New England Journal of Medicine* 1994; **331**: 1416–20.

9. Thomsen HS. Contrast nephrotoxicity. In: Willi U, Kenney PJ, Thomsen HS, eds. *International Uroradiology '96*. Copenhagen: FADL Publishers, 1996: 160–7.

Case studies: urgent decisions in interventional radiology

Michael A. Bettmann

Introduction

Interventional radiology is playing an increasingly important role in patient care. Its efficacy is widely accepted, and there is a low incidence of complications with most procedures. None the less, complications clearly do occur, and it is imperative that all medical personnel who deal with interventional radiology are aware of what can go wrong, how to prevent complications, and how to treat them should they arise.

The following case presentations are designed to review some of the scenarios that may be encountered during interventional procedures.

Case studies

Case 1

A 68-year-old woman presented to the Cardiovascular and Interventional Radiology Section with a diagnosis of hypertension and a duplex ultrasound study which suggested left renal artery stenosis. Her past medical history was significant for a myocardial infarction 4 years previously, class II angina and a history of 100 pack-years of smoking. She was on three medications for her hypertension, which was still not considered to be controlled optimally. On examination, the patient had a blood pressure of 160/100 mmHg in the right arm and 165/110 mmHg in the left arm. Femoral pulses were present, although they were slightly diminished on the left. The patient underwent an arteriogram utilizing the right percutaneous femoral approach. A sheath was placed in the groin and an abdominal aortogram was performed which showed moderate diffuse atherosclerosis, non-significant stenosis diffusely in a single right renal artery and two left renal arteries. The left superior polar artery was relatively small. The medium-sized left main renal artery had a significant proximal, non-ostial stenosis.

Because of the hypertension and this significant left stenosis, it was decided to angioplasty and stent this proximal lesion. The lesion was predilated with a 6-mm balloon, and a stent was then placed and deployed with a 7-mm balloon. After the angioplasty, the angiographic appearance was good, with moderate irregularity remaining but no significant stenosis. The patient was stable, and the catheter was removed with good hemostasis.

Approximately 15 min later, the patient's blood pressure was noted to be 100/60 mmHg with a heart rate of 70 beats/min. She complained of nausea and vomited once. She also complained of mild back pain. What is happening in this patient, and what should be done?

Possible responses

(a) The patient is having a vasovagal reaction. Give fluids, elevate the legs and give 0.5–1.0 mg of atropine intravenously.
(b) This is an expected response to an acute change in renal flow. Nothing needs to be done other than observation.
(c) This is a contrast reaction. It is likely to resolve spontaneously and nothing needs to be done.
(d) There may be a rupture of the renal artery. The patient should be observed very carefully and, if necessary, CT possibly followed by repeat angiography should be considered.

Discussion

(a) Vasovagal reactions are fairly common and may occur not only during but also following a procedure, particularly during painful compression following removal of a catheter. Although usually accompanied by bradycardia and hypotension, there can occasionally be a stable heart rate, or merely the absence of tachycardia. Vasovagal reactions are often heralded by nausea and vomiting. Treatment with fluids (given carefully in this patient with known coronary artery disease), leg elevation, and even atropine at a dose of 0.5–1.0 mg is a reasonable first step. However, the patient should be carefully observed. The renal artery intervention combined with back pain should raise a suspicion that this is not merely a vasovagal response.

(b) Blood pressure can fall rapidly after renal angioplasty. Particular care must be taken in patients who remain on antihypertensive medications immediately prior to the procedure. However, it is unusual for postangioplasty hypotension to be accompanied by other symptoms, such as nausea and vomiting or back pain. It is also rather unusual for the pressure to fall to below normal levels, despite antihypertensive medications. Such a fall may occur as the patient stands up, but this patient's hypotension was not postural.

(c) Delayed contrast reactions can occur, but are generally cutaneous in nature. Hypotension, minor tachycardia and back pain in this patient suggest that this is not a contrast reaction.

(d) In this patient with known atherosclerosis and a relatively small renal artery that was dilated (since there are two left renal arteries), plus symptoms which hint at a retroperitoneal process, it is important to consider the possibility of renal artery rupture. This is an infrequent but known complication of renal angioplasty and stenting. Such a rupture is generally contained and self-limiting. None the less, careful evaluation is mandatory. In this situation, with marginal blood pressure and without marked tachycardia, it is reasonable to observe vital signs frequently and cautiously, give IV fluids and treat initially with atropine. As with most patients on multiple medications for control of hypertension, one of this patient's medicines was a beta-blocker. This explains the absence of tachycardia. It is also reasonable to perform a CT scan without oral or IV contrast in order to assess whether there is substantial retroperitoneal bleeding. Although, it would be possible to re-engage the renal artery with an angiographic catheter and put in another stent to help to block a leak, this is rarely necessary. Another option for such a patient who becomes profoundly hypotensive is to inflate a balloon catheter in the renal artery. The patient can then be taken to surgery for ligation of the renal artery and placement of a bypass graft. Alternatively, if this artery supplies a relatively small portion of the two kidneys and if renal function is normal, or if the patient is at high operative risk, infusion of absolute alcohol to ablate this portion of the kidney is a possibility. This leads to cessation of inflow and is another way of controlling bleeding. A crucial point to remember in this situation is that the balloon and/or stent that were used may have been slightly oversized for this situation, as this artery was one of two left renal arteries in a woman. As with all such situations, close observation and continual evaluation are imperative until it is clear that the patient is stable.

Answer   (a) and (d)

Case 2
A 71-year-old man presented with a history of recent onset of shortness of breath and pleuritic chest pain after relative bedrest since a myocardial infarction 2 weeks previously. Because of the suspicion of pulmonary embolism, the patient underwent ultrasound studies of the lower extremities and the findings were equivocal. A chest X-ray showed minor bibasilar atelectasis and a ventilation-perfusion lung scan showed several subsegmental defects and bibasilar matched segmental perfusion-ventilation defects. The scan was therefore interpreted as low-intermediate probability. Because of the relatively high clinical suspicion and lack of confirmation from non-invasive studies, pulmonary angiography was requested.

A pulmonary angiogram was performed from the right percutaneous femoral venous approach. A pigtail catheter and guidewire were advanced into the right atrium. The mean pressure in the right atrium was 14 mmHg. As the catheter was advanced over the guidewire into the right ventricle, the patient began to have ventricular premature contractions.

Possible responses

(a) Pull the catheter out, terminate the procedure and suggest CT for evaluation of possible pulmonary emboli.

(b) Ignore ventricular ectopy and continue the procedure.

(c) Pull the catheter out, request that a cardiologist come to the interventional/angiography suite and then proceed only with a cardiologist in attendance and/or with a pacemaker in place.

(d) Reposition the catheter and guidewire and continue with the procedure.

Discussion   It is very common for ectopy to occur during pulmonary angiography as the right ventricle is traversed with the guidewire and catheter, due to the irritability of this chamber. This is particularly troublesome in certain patients, such as those who are recently post myocardial infarction (MI), have had recent cardiac surgery, have underlying arrhythmias or have a left bundle branch block. These arrhythmias generally consist of runs of premature ventricular contractions (PVCs). They almost always stop when the catheter and guidewire are removed from the right ventricle, or when the right ventricle is traversed and the catheter and guidewire lie in the pulmonary artery. Great care must be taken in all patients to ensure that the catheter is not positioned so as to allow the arrhythmias to persist. Some angiographers are careful to have a transcutaneous pacemaker or a transvenous pacing wire available in the case of patients with a history of arrhythmias, particularly those with left bundle branch block. No other specific precautions are necessary.

In general, arrhythmias such as PVCs are expected, but careful surveillance is necessary to ensure that they are infrequent or that runs of PVCs are brief. If more than a few occur, the catheter and wire should be rapidly removed from the ventricle. A different catheter/guidewire combination or a different angle can then be attempted for catheterization of the pulmonary artery. One should have the necessary equipment and knowledge to deal with a full cardiopulmonary arrest; a cardiologist consultation, a pacing wire or a Code are rarely necessary in this situation.

Answer   (d)

Case 3

A 49-year-old man presented with a history of increasing scleral icterus over the last few months. He had noted minor weight loss and a change in stool color, but no other symptoms or signs. Abdominal ultrasound suggested a pancreatic mass. Endoscopic retrograde cholangiopancreatography (ERCP) showed an obstructed common bile duct, but the duct could not be entered from below. A percutaneous cholangiogram with drainage was therefore requested.

Under local anesthesia with intravenous sedation, a percutaneous cholangiogram was performed from the right lateral approach with a 21-gauge needle.

Obstruction of the mid common bile duct was confirmed, with marked biliary dilatation intrahepatically. Subsequently, the bile duct was entered with a needle-and-wire combination, a catheter was manipulated through the obstruction, the obstruction was dilated sequentially, and a 10-Fr. internal–external drainage tube was placed with side holes both above and below the obstruction. The patient tolerated this procedure well initially, with pain that was readily controlled, and the catheter was left to external drainage. Within minutes, however, drainage was noted to change from pure bile to blood-tinged bile. During the ensuing 15 min, approximately 300 mL of blood/bile drained out. The patient's blood pressure at the start of the procedure had been 145/85mmHg. During the procedure, with sedation, the blood pressure fell slightly, to 130/70mmHg. Now the patient had no significant tachycardia, but the pressure was slightly lower still, at 110/60 mmHg. At this point the patient was awake and alert without complaints except for mild tenderness at the puncture site.

Possible responses

(a) Cap the drainage tube and allow the patient to drain internally, assuming that the bleeding is minor and will be self-contained.

(b) Perform an arteriogram to document whether or not the patient has a focal arterial bleeding site and treat accordingly.

(c) Assume that the bleeding is venous in origin and allow the patient to drain externally, assuming that he can be carefully monitored and fluid and blood replaced as needed.

(d) Perform an abdominal CT to look for subcapsular or intraperitoneal bleeding. If any is present, call for a surgeon for consultation.

Discussion   Although the initial blood loss via the drainage tube was relatively small, it can be assumed that the patient was also bleeding through the tube and into the bowel. The gradual downward drift in blood pressure is a worrying sign. Watchful waiting, with the tube either capped or uncapped, is probably not indicated at this point. Further assessment by CT with possible surgery is also unlikely to be helpful. Surgical intervention in this setting is likely to be very difficult, as the bleeding site is probably intrahepatic and will be difficult to identify at the time of operation. If the blood loss appears to be continuing, as reflected by blood in the drainage tube and by hypotension with or without tachycardia, it is distinctly possible that a hepatic artery branch has been traversed during the procedure and is the source of bleeding. Venous bleeding from either the portal or hepatic venous circulations is generally minor, and tends to stop spontaneously and fairly quickly. In order to document and treat a hepatic arterial bleeding site, selective angiography is necessary.

A catheter should be placed into the hepatic artery and injections made. If no obvious bleeding site is seen, it is wise to remove the drainage catheter, leaving a guidewire in place, and then to repeat the hepatic angiogram (to eliminate the possibility that the bleeding is being partially tamponaded by the catheter). If the bleeding site is identified, it should be treated by embolization, and coils are particularly useful in this setting. This is a known but relatively infrequent complication of biliary drainage procedures. Such bleeding may occur in a delayed manner. Embolization, usually with a coil, is curative in this situation.

Answer   (b)

Case 4

A 59-year-old man presented with worsening left leg claudication. The patient had a history of claudication for the past 2 years, progressing from approximately 300 yards to less than 50 yards. He had no history of other cardiovascular disease. His serum cholesterol had been noted to be mildly elevated, but he received no treatment for this, apart from the suggestion of a low-fat diet. He had a history of 80 pack-years of cigarette smoking. Serum creatinine, prothrombin time (PT) and partial thromboplastin time (PTT) were all within normal limits. The patient was referred for angiography, and an initial evaluation demonstrated a normal right femoral pulse with a moderately diminished left femoral pulse. The ankle-brachial artery index was 0.85 on the right and 0.55 on the left. Angiography was performed utilizing the left percutaneous femoral approach. This showed moderate atherosclerotic disease in the aorta, moderate diffuse disease in the right iliac system, a normal left common iliac artery and a 75 per cent stenosis over approximately 2 cm in the left external iliac artery. Moderate disease was seen more distally, with one vessel runoff bilaterally.

Angioplasty was considered, with the plan that a stent would be placed if the angioplasty was not satisfactory. The normal portion of the left external iliac artery was measured, and the diameter was thought to be 6 mm. A 7-mm-diameter × 2-cm-long balloon was chosen. This was inflated to 8 atmospheres of pressure in the left external iliac artery. After a 1-min inflation, a repeat angiogram showed a dissection involving the segment that was angioplastied. Although flow was good, the decision was made to use a larger balloon to treat this dissection. An 8 mm × 2-cm balloon catheter was inflated, again at 8 atmospheres, for 1 min. After deflation, the patient's blood pressure had fallen from a peak systolic pressure of 150 mmHg to a systolic pressure of 80 mmHg. His heart rate had risen from 80 to 110 beats/min. A hand injection of contrast showed extravasation at the angioplasty site.

Possible responses

(a) Call a vascular surgeon and send the patient to the operating room (OR) immediately.

(b) Place an 8-mm diameter × 4-cm-long stent across the area of extravasation.

(c) Reinflate the original 8-mm balloon catheter high in the external iliac artery and alert the vascular surgery department to the need for emergent bypass.

(d) Place a stent across the area of extravasation, reinflate an 8-mm balloon above the stented area, and reassess after 10–20 min.

Discussion   The first consideration in this patient is to control the rapid blood loss due to rupture of the external iliac artery. This can generally be achieved most rapidly and effectively by reinflating the balloon above the site of the rupture. Simultaneously, the vascular surgery department should be notified that the patient will probably need emergent bypass. If a covered stent is available, consideration can be given to placing it. This is a method that clearly works, but such stents are not yet widely available commercially. Placing an uncovered stent, if there is frank extravasation, is unlikely to be helpful. It also has the drawback of possibly making surgical access to this site more difficult. If there is merely intravasation of contrast into the wall, which is not an unusual occurrence, there is generally little blood loss and the patient would not have tachycardia and hypotension. However, in the presence of the progressing symptoms it is unlikely that either placing an uncovered stent or inflating a balloon and waiting will lead to satisfactory control of the vessel leak. Although a pinpoint rupture is a distinct possibility, a larger rupture is more likely to have occurred, and this will always need definitive repair. Such a repair should not be delayed. Conversely, it is imperative that the bleeding be controlled as rapidly as possible to prevent further, potentially life-endangering blood loss while the patient is waiting for surgery, and this can be achieved with the balloon catheter.

Answer   (c)

Case 5

A 46-year-old woman presented with a history of 5 years of hypertension with recent marked worsening and difficulty in achieving adequate control. Renal duplex ultrasound suggested left renal artery stenosis, and the patient was referred for angiographic evaluation and treatment. The patient had a history of long-term tobacco use and a strong family history of early atherosclerosis. Her father died at the age of 45 years following a myocardial infarction, two brothers had myocardial infarctions in their forties, and the patient's mother died of a cerebrovascular accident (CVA) at the age of 65 years. The patient had normal serum cholesterol and no history of other cardiovascular disease. Her serum creatinine level was 1.1 mg/dL and bleeding parameters were normal.

The patient underwent a diagnostic arteriogram using the right percutaneous femoral approach. The aortogram showed a tight left renal artery stenosis. A 7-Fr. sheath was placed in the right groin, the renal artery lesion was crossed with a steerable guidewire, 5000 units of heparin were administered and the lesion was dilated and stented with a 1.5-cm-length × 6-mm-diameter stent. Following the procedure, the catheter and guidewire were removed. The activated clotting time (ACT) was measured and the initial reading was 225 s. On remeasurement 90 min later, the ACT had decreased to a level of 160 s and the sheath was removed without incident. A small hematoma was noted prior to the patient's discharge. The next day, the patient called to say that she had no bleeding or other problems, her blood pressure was normal on no medication, but that she had a swelling in her groin at the site of the arterial puncture which was pulsatile and slightly tender. She thought that it was larger than it had been at the time of discharge.

Possible responses

    (a) Refer the patient to the vascular surgery department for evaluation of a possible arterial injury.

    (b) Reassure the patient that this is not a major cause for concern. Encourage her to call back if the hematoma enlarges in size or if the tenderness persists over the next 4–7 days.

    (c) Perform an angiogram, utilizing another access site, to assess the arterial injury.

    (d) Ask the patient to come in and then evaluate this area with ultrasound, to exclude the possibility of a pseudoaneurysm.

Discussion   Hematomas are relatively common following interventional procedures. Although data are relatively sparse, it is logical to assume that the incidence and severity of hematomas increase with increasing catheter size and with use of anticoagulation therapy. There is no evidence to support the idea that the incidence or severity increase with the use of antiplatelet therapy, such as aspirin or ticlopidine. Most hematomas are self-limiting and of no consequence. Hematomas can occasionally (but rarely) be large enough to require blood transfusions, and sometimes they may be related to inadvertent puncture of the femoral artery above the inguinal ligament, with retroperitoneal bleeding. This is generally also self-limiting, but may require surgical repair.

Perhaps the most frequent significant complication of arterial access at the groin is the formation of a pseudoaneurysm. The incidence is unknown, but their occurrence is well documented. In the past, pseudoaneurysms have been regarded as a surgical emergency, as they can rupture and cause life-threatening bleeding. Over the last few years, extensive experience has been gained in 'repairing' pseudoaneurysms by compression, while monitoring with the ultrasound probe. This treatment is almost always effective, with a low incidence of complications or recurrence. Furthermore, it is clear from experience with ultrasound compression that pseudoaneurysms are not true emergencies. Although urgent treatment is a reasonable approach, it is safe to wait for 12–24 h before instituting ultrasound evaluation and compression. Vascular surgical repair, either before or after ultrasound compression, is rarely if ever necessary. In general, it is important to assess any unusual hematomas to ensure that they are simply hematomas and not pseudoaneurysms. Most, but not all, occur in patients who have had relatively large sheaths placed and have had high levels of anticoagulation therapy during the procedure. They are most likely to form in patients with moderate to large hematomas.

Answer   (d)

Case 6

A 63-year-old white man with a fever of unknown origin for the past 6 weeks, a history of frequent travel to various Asian countries, and 30 pack-years of smoking presented with a solitary lung nodule. Aspiration biopsy for cytology and culture was requested. The patient was otherwise in good health. Clotting parameters were normal. The patient was put on the fluoroscopy table, and a peripheral IV was started, sedation was given and an access site was documented, with fluoroscopy, on the right anterior chest wall. Xylocaine was infused intradermally, a small incision was made and an 18-gauge biopsy needle was advanced under fluoroscopic control. Immediately after the first aspiration, the patient complained of nausea. He was noted to be somewhat diaphoretic and he mentioned that he felt lightheaded.

Possible responses

(a) The patient may have developed a pneumothorax during the first needle pass. An erect chest film should be obtained. If a pneumothorax is present, a small-bore chest tube should be placed.

(b) Reassure the patient that this is a common reaction. Assess the sample, and take another sample if necessary.

(c) Give additional sedation and proceed as indicated, based on the adequacy of the first sample.

(d) Assess the patient's vital signs. If he is hypotensive and bradycardic, elevate his legs, start to administer fluids and consider further medications, specifically atropine, as necessary.

Discussion   A pneumothorax following a lung biopsy is a well-known occurrence. The incidence is as high as 20–30 per cent, and is a function of the location of the lesion (pleural based vs. central), needle size and number of needle passes. In general, such pneumothoraces are either asymptomatic or present with pleuritic chest pain, occasionally accompanied by dyspnea and/or hypoxia. They can often be assessed with fluoroscopy, but an upright chest film may be required. A chest tube is sometimes indicated and, if so, a small-bore (8-Fr.) pigtail-shaped catheter can be placed and left to suction or even to a unidirectional Heimlich valve. In our experience, a small catheter placed laterally in the mid-axillary or anterior-axillary line is more effective than one in the mid-clavicular line. It is equivalent to a large chest tube.

Vasovagal reactions can occur with any intervention. They clearly occur after the injection of contrast agents, but they also arise in response to needle sticks or even to anxiety alone. They are often heralded clinically by nausea, diaphoresis and lightheadedness. In any situation in which the patient is experiencing a reaction, vital signs should be obtained. If the patient is hypotensive and bradycardic, or even shows hypotension and a lack of tachycardia, a vasovagal reaction is the likely explanation. The first treatment for this is leg elevation and fluids. It is important to ensure that the vasovagal reaction resolves completely. This may require the use of atropine at a minimal dose of 0.5 mg IV. If appropriately treated with leg elevation, volume expansion and atropine, vasovagal reactions generally always resolve. However, if left untreated they can progress rapidly to more severe, life-threatening reactions, complicated by arrhythmias and worse. It is therefore important to assess all such reactions fully, and to follow patients carefully in order to ensure that the reaction (specifically the hypotension and bradycardia) resolve completely.

Answer   (d), then (a)

Appendices

Appendix I: Premedication protocols

Option 1: Corticosteroid plus antihistamine
Prednisone 50 mg by mouth at 13, 7 and 1 h before contrast medium injection
Diphenhydramine 50 mg by mouth or IM 1 h before contrast medium injection

Option 2: Corticosteroid
Methylprednisolone 32 mg by mouth at 12 and 2 h before contrast medium injection

Option 3: Urgent situation
Hydrocortisone 100 mg IV at 4–6 h and 1 h before contrast medium injection
Diphenhydramine 50 mg (orally, IV or IM) 1 h before contrast medium injection

Appendix II: Treatment outline for contrast reactions in adults

Hypotension (isolated)
Elevate patient's legs
Oxygen by mask (10 L/min)
IV isotonic fluids (primary therapy)
If unresponsive, administer vasopressor, e.g. epinephrine IV

Vagal reaction (hypotension and bradycardia)
Elevate patient's legs
Oxygen by mask (10 L/min)
IV isotonic fluids
Atropine, 1.0 mg IV, repeat as necessary to 0.04mg/kg total dose

Bronchospasm (isolated)
Oxygen by mask (6–10 L/min)
Beta-2-agonist metered-dose inhaler
Epinephrine:
  normal blood pressure, stable bronchospasm:
    Subcutaneous, 1:1000 0.1–0.2 mL (0.1–0.2 mg)

Progressive bronchospasm and/or decreased blood pressure:
IV, 1:10 000 dilution, 1 mL (0.1 mg), slowly over 2–5 min,
repeat or increase dose rate as necessary

Laryngeal edema
Oxygen by mask (10 L/min)
Epinephrine (1:10 000), IV, 1 ml (0.1mg) slowly over 2–5 min,
repeat or increase dose rate as needed

Anaphylactoid reaction (generalized systemic reaction)
Suction as necessary
Elevate patient's legs if hypotensive
Oxygen by mask (10 L/min)
IV isotonic fluids
Epinephrine:
IV: 1:10 000 dilution, 1 mL (0.1 mg) slowly (e.g. incrementally over 2–5
min); repeat or increase dose rate as needed
Beta-2-agonist metered-dose inhaler
Antihistamines:
H-1 antihistamine and H-2 antihistamine
Corticosteroids:
hydrocortisone 250–500 mg IV; methylprednisolone 40–80 mg IV

Urticaria
Mild: observation
H-1 antihistamine
Severe: *add*
IV fluids (isotonic)
Epinephrine (1:10 000 dilution) IV, 1 mL (0.1 mg) slowly
H-2 antihistamine

Angina
Oxygen by mask (10 L/min)
IV access, fluids very slowly
Nitroglycerin: 0.4 mg sublingually, may repeat after 5–15 min

Hypertension
Oxygen by mask (10 L/min)
IV access, fluids very slowly
Nitroglycerin:
orally (sublingually), 0.4 mg tablet or sublingual spray; IV: 100–200 μg
topically, 2 per cent ointment: apply 1–2 inch strip to skin
If secondary to autonomic dysreflexia: nifedipine, 10 mg capsule, punctured or
chewed and contents swallowed;
If secondary to pheochromocytoma: phentolamine, 5 mg, IV slowly

Seizures

Protect the patient
Airway: suction as necessary; monitor airway for obstruction by tongue
Oxygen by mask (10 L/min)
If caused by hypotension with or without bradycardia, treat as per protocol.
Uncontrolled: diazepam, 5 mg, IV

Appendix III: Treatment outline for contrast reactions in children

Vagal reaction (hypotension and bradycardia)

Oxygen by mask
IV fluids
Atropine: 0.02 mg/kg IV; min. initial dose 0.1 mg, max. initial dose 0.6 mg

Bronchospasm (isolated)

Oxygen by mask
Beta-2-agonist metered-dose inhaler
Epinephrine:
  Normal blood pressure, stable bronchospasm:
    Subcutaneous: 1:1000 dilution, 0.01 mg/kg up to 0.3 mg maximum
  Progressive bronchospasm and/or decreased blood pressure:
    IV: 1:10 000 dilution, 0.01 mg/kg to 0.1 mg max.

Laryngeal edema and/or generalized systemic reaction

Suction as necessary
Oxygen by mask
Epinephrine: IV: 1:10 000 dilution, 0.01 mg/kg, to 0.1 mg

Appendix IV: Drugs and medications for Rad-LS treatment kit

Drug	Amount
Atropine, 1 mg	3
(1-mg ampoule or prepackaged solution)	
Beta-2 agonist metered-dose inhaler	1
(e.g. metaproterenol)	
Epinephrine, 1:1000 dilution	1
(1 mg ampoule)	
Epinephrine, 1:10 000 dilution	1
(prepackaged dilution of 1 mg)	
H-1 antihistamine	1
(e.g. diphenhydramine for injection, 50 mg)	
H-2 antihistamine	1
(e.g. cimetidine for injection, 300 mg)	

Nitroglycerin   1
    (e.g. bottle of 0.4-mg oral tablets or tube of 2 per cent topical ointment)
Nifedepine   1
    (e.g. 10-mg gelatin capsule)
Corticosteroid   1
    (e.g. hydrocortisone 250 or 500 mg or methylprednisolone 80 mg for
      injection)

Optional drugs and medications

Beta agonist   1
    (e.g. isoproterenol 0.2 mg for injection)
Dextrose 50 per cent solution   1
    (e.g. 25 g in prepackaged syringe)
Diuretic   1
    (e.g. furosemide, 40 mg for injection)
Intravenous fluids, 500 or 1000 mL   1
    (0.9 per cent saline or lactated Ringer's solution)

Additional equipment

Alcohol wipes
Blood-pressure cuff
IV catheters
IV tubing
One-way mouth-to-mask resuscitation device
Oral airways (adult and pediatric)
Stethoscope
Syringes
Tape
Tourniquet

Index